Ready, Set, GO!

SYNERGY FITNESS

for Time-Crunched Adults

Phil Campbell, M.S., M.A., FACHE

First Edition 2002

Pristine Publishers Inc. USA

Published by:
Pristine Publishers Inc. USA
ISBN 0-9716633-9-4
www.readysetgofitness.com
E-mail: pristine@charter.net

    This book is designed to provide information in regard to the subject matter covered for healthy adults. It is sold with the understanding that the publisher, author and advisors are not rendering medical advice or other professional services. It is highly recommended that an examination by a physician be performed BEFORE attempting to begin any fitness training programs outlined in this book.

    The purpose of this book is to educate, expand thinking about fitness as an informational source for readers, and it is not medical advice, nor has it been evaluated by the FDA. The publisher, author, and advisors shall have neither liability nor responsibility to any person or entity with respect to any loss or damage caused or alleged to be caused directly or indirectly by the information and programs contained in this book. If you do not agree with the above, you may return to the publisher for a full refund.

FIRST EDITION 2002

Printed in USA by Vaughan Printing, Nashville
Designed by Bruce Gore, Gore Studios, Nashville
Layout by Maria C. Hasz, Jackson, TN

Library of Congress Card Number 2001135854

ISBN 0-9716633-9-4

Contents

About the Author

Phil Campbell wrote his first fitness training manual over 30 years ago. While in college, he managed health clubs and

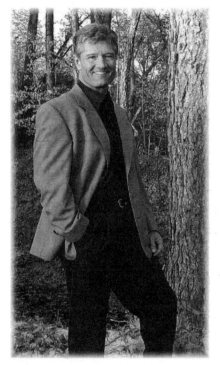 performed personal training 20 years before it was called personal training.

Two masters degrees later, and a 20-year career as a healthcare executive that included serving as a Division President with eight hospitals under his command, he returned to writing about fitness, improving athletic performance, anti-aging, and anti Middle-aging.

He's been nicknamed the "anti Middle-aging guy."

Age 50

Phil Campbell will be 50 on his next birthday. He shares his unique experience of how a 20-year career healthcare executive and a father of three can achieve optimum fitness improvement as a time-crunched adult.

With years of experience in taking complex medical subjects and making them understandable and practical, he has written a complete guide—based on the latest discoveries in medical research—that shows readers step-by-step how to improve fitness, energy, and appearance.

Phil Campbell is the creator of **Synergy Fitness**—a comprehensive fitness training approach targeted at five major areas of fitness—flexibility, endurance, strength, power, and anaerobic conditioning.

As a masters athlete, Phil Campbell holds several USA Track and Field Masters titles including first place in the 100-meter sprint, Southeastern U.S. Championships for his age group in 2000. In 2001, he placed third nationally in USA Track and Field Masters Nationals in his age group in the javelin throw, fifth in discus, and he won medals in several 100 and 200 meter sprint competitions. In his late 40s, he won a 40-yard dash competition in 4.69 seconds. He has a black belt in Isshinryu Karate, and has competed and won first place in marital arts and weightlifting competitions.

Phil Campbell will show you how to have the most successful—and lasting—fitness improvement experience of your life.

What Others are Saying About this Book...

Alvin Hoover,
Hospital administrator

"The next fitness revolution is here and it's called *Synergy Fitness*. I was finishing my masters in Exercise Science when *Aerobics* fired the shot that started the world running and ushered in the "Cardio" revolution. *Synergy Fitness* is destined to change fitness training as we know it today."

Detective Captain Mickey Miller,
Metropolitan Nashville Police

"Phil Campbell has discovered the secret to maximizing exercise potential. His book does it all. Phil provides the most comprehensive exercise plans I have seen to date. And I have tried virtually every type of program that has come out in the past 30 years.

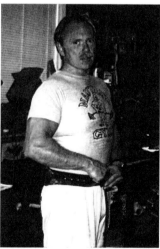

It seemed that as I got older, positive results were impossible to achieve, impossible that is, until I began following the step-by-step programs developed by Phil Campbell. This program has changed my life both physically and mentally for the good. Thanks Phil."

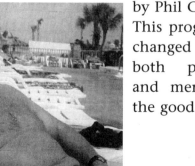

Mickey 90 days after starting Synergy Fitness

May 2001, one week before starting Synergy Fitness

Dr. Keith Williams, Ob-Gyn

"As a physician, I recognize and encourage patients in the importance of exercise and nutrition and the benefits obtained from a sustained program. But like most, I struggle with the ability to maintain an exercise program. For two decades I have tried multiple programs but have been frustrated by the time commitment, expense, isolated results, and lack of desired results for maintaining overall physical health.

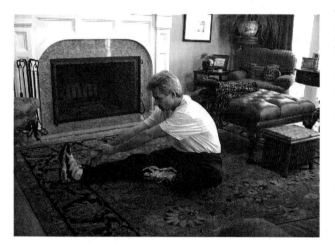

Dr. Williams performing the 10-Minute Stretching Routine

After reading Phil's book, I started the Synergy Fitness program. I was amazed at the results I achieved in body flexibility, strength, endurance, and improvement in overall sense of well being that results from a regular exercise program. Most of all I was able to accomplish this with a reasonable time investment, because I was able to do the program on my time at home.

Phil's plan is practical, scientifically based, and meets my goals for good health now and into the future."

Nan Allison, MS, RD, Licensed Nutritionist Author of *Full and Fulfilled*

"Very convincing....and it works! This is a well researched and clearly presented case for naturally increasing your Human Growth Hormone. Not only that, Phil Campbell, tells you how to do it, simply. I now understand why even the best diet, long walks and regular weight lifting weren't giving me the same benefits as I thought they should. With a few tweaks to my workout program (and no more time involvement), I have twice the energy and feel more toned than I've felt in a long time. Read this book and you'll understand why."

Dr. Larry Schrader
Orthopedic Surgeon

"I have known Phil, professionally and as a training partner, for several years. He was able to rekindle my interest in competitive athletics after a 20 year lay off. I was recently able to win Master's National Titles in both powerlifting and Track and Field. Phil has also taken the lead in training techniques, general fitness and nutrition.

I practice orthopedic surgery including sports medicine and muscle and joint reconstruction. Phil has thoughtfully gathered the cutting edge thinking regarding strength, flexibility and nutrition which can enable all of us to participate in athletics our entire lives and maybe even exceed the accomplishments of our youth. This is a doable program for a tight schedule and can keep you energized as well as injury free and competitive."

Dr. Keith Atkins
Internal Medicine, Specialist

"I personally follow the Synergy Fitness Plan and recommend it to all my patients."

Acknowledgments

It is an honor to recognize, and publicly thank key individuals who contributed to the creation, development and production of this book.

From the initial encouragement to write this book, to taking all photo illustrations, to proofreading text, I must first thank my wife, Kathy, for her contributions and commitment to this project. Thanks to my children Holly, Christine and John for serving as Synergy Fitness demonstrators and reminding me of the really important things in life. And thanks to my mom, Bertha McClenny, for her unconditional love and support.

I am indebted to many for their contributions; Bruce Gore, Gore Studios for book cover and interior design; Mary Sanford for editing; and proofreaders Dr. Lorraine Singer, Pat Thomson, and Maria Hasz who patiently placed the text and photo illustrations into the book.

In addition, I want to thank literary attorney and author Lee Wilson for her advice; and authors Nan Allison and Pat Winston for their coaching. Many thanks to my wife's training partners, certified personal trainers Bambi LaFont and Melanie Joyner for illustrating Synergy Fitness techniques. Also, thanks to everyone who helped demonstrate training techniques for the book.

Special thanks to my training partners–Nate Robertson, Dr. Larry Schrader, Terry Bumpus, and my track coach Wes Reade for his information and motivation; Jon and Susan Parrish, owners of Lord's Gym; and the others who assisted with this book.

Lastly, I dedicate this book to biomedical researchers. Sometimes they are listed in bibliographies tucked in the back of books. Seldom do they receive the recognition they deserve for the enormous impact they have on the lives of others.

Welcome To Synergy Fitness

What is Synergy Fitness?

Synergy Fitness is a set of ten strategies based on current medical research (with no gimmicks, no fluff) to lead you to the highest level of fitness possible—in the shortest amount of time.

The **Ten Synergy Fitness Strategies** will help you lose weight, tone and build muscle, increase energy, delay the effects of aging—and middle aging—improve appearance, and improve athletic performance.

Synergy Fitness Has Three Main Goals

• **Synergy Fitness** shows you how to increase key hormones in your body naturally (athletic performance improving, anti-aging, and anti–middle aging hormones) while you exercise—so your body will continue to tone, add muscle, and burn fat for up to three hours after you finish training.

Some athletes take hormone injections to improve performance. And several well-known actors report that they take hormone injections to look and feel 20 years younger—this book shows you how to increase these same hormones naturally.

• **Synergy Fitness** shows you how to combine several forms of exercise (multi-tasking) to increase results and save time. By offering comprehensive, pre-designed, Strategic Fitness Plans for time-crunched adults–in an easy-to-follow format–you can obtain maximum benefits in the shortest amount of time. And Synergy Fitness offers five different plans that are based on age, current fitness status, and training experience.   So beginners, all the way to professional athletes, will have a plan to meet their needs.

• **Synergy Fitness** seeks to provide you with the most exciting, productive fitness improvement experience of your life—that will last a lifetime.

What Is Synergy?

Synergy is the perfect term to describe the health and fitness impact of increasing key hormones in your body. It means, literally, combining two or more parts together. And because the parts are acting together, rather than separately, the total outcome is greater than the sum of the individual parts.

Achieving great results in the shortest amount of time possible is what Synergy Fitness is all about.

Sections in This Book

Synergy Fitness for Time-Crunched Adults sticks to its philosophy: cut through the gimmicks (quickly) and deliver. Deliver real information that you can begin using immediately. Synergy Fitness will bring you all the excitement and action of a race.

Just before the race begins, you hear the loud words: "Ready" . . . "Set." And on "GO!" the action explodes. This book follows that same course. The first two sections of the book prepare you for the greatest fitness improvement experience of your life. The information in these sections will have you **Ready** and **Set** to implement the **Ten Synergy Fitness Strategies** in the **GO** section.

HELPFUL INFORMATION: As you go through this book, you will see shaded boxes like this that contain supporting medical research. These boxes allow you to see the reliability of the information and the date of the scientific research.

My Promise: "No Wasted Time, No Gimmicks, No Fluff!"

If you are a time-crunched adult like me, you probably thumb through magazines and books to determine if the information is worth reading. Let me assure you—the time you spend with this book will yield significant health, fitness, appearance, and energy dividends. However, before the race begins, there is the necessary *Ready* and *Set* preparation time.

Chapters 1–10 are packed with information to help you—whatever your age or current fitness condition— achieve exciting new levels of fitness. Let me encourage you not to jump to the *GO* phase without first going through the *Ready* and *Set* phases. You'll miss some great information if you do!

The New England Journal of Medicine published a study showing growth hormone replacement therapy increased muscle mass by 8.8 percent and decreased fat by 14.4 percent in older adults. (Rudman).

Why Are Famous Actors, Athletes, and Bodybuilders Taking Hormones?

Recent discoveries about hormones, particularly growth hormone (GH), are changing the way scientists think about fitness, health, athletic performance, aging, and even middle aging. The benefits of the research discoveries apply to athletes of all ages, patients at anti-aging centers, and middle-aged adults trying to lose weight, get in shape, and restore the energy of their youth.

Children with severe growth problems have been treated with growth hormone effectively for years; it makes them grow taller and stronger. Growth hormone will not make adults grow taller. Researchers show that increasing growth hormone in adults will tone and build muscle, drop body fat significantly, increase energy, and make adults younger in appearance.

From *USA Today* to *Oprah*, the miraculous benefits of increasing growth hormone have been touted, and rightfully so—the benefits of increasing growth hormone are almost miraculous!

And new medical research shows that growth hormone *can* be increased naturally. Specific types of fitness training, adequate "slow wave" deep sleep, and select nutritional supplements have been shown in recent biomedical research studies to increase the body's natural release of growth hormone.

Increasing growth hormone (GH) improves athletic performance. Olympians and bodybuilders attempting to improve athletic performance and muscular appearance have been reported to use growth hormone injections—a banned substance for athletes because it improves performance. Worldwide headlines focused on the abuse of growth hormone and steroids by Olympians during the 2000 Games.

Medical researchers, attempting to delay the effects of aging, treated adults with the same GH therapy used for treating children. The results were phenomenal. Increasing growth hormone in adults was found to reverse the effects of aging—equivalent to 10 to 20 years of aging.

And today, some biomedical researchers are debating the idea of delaying "somatopause" (so-MOT-a-pause)—the metabolism slow-down, weight gain phase of middle age—with growth hormone therapy.

The key question is—what if there's a way to get the benefits of GH therapy—without injections—naturally? That's what this book is about! Growth hormone can be increased naturally. And this book will show you how to do it!

The discovery that GH can be increased naturally will revolutionize the health and fitness world during the next decade. You can get so much more than the calorie burning benefits of exercise by performing the type of fitness training that increases your body's natural release of GH. There is real fitness synergy available with specific types of exercise, as you will see as you read this book.

There is no need for potentially harmful GH injections for most adults. With the correct Strategic Fitness Plan, aimed at increasing GH in your body naturally, you can significantly improve fitness, health, appearance, and energy, lose weight, tone and build muscle, and feel great! And that is the ultimate purpose of this book—to provide you with a precise plan for how you can receive the synergistic benefits of naturally increasing growth hormone in your body.

Exercise has a profound effect on the release of growth hormone. (Growth hormone and exercise, 1999, Jenkins).

Based on Medical Research

Ready, Set, GO! Synergy Fitness for Time-Crunched Adults presents discoveries by biomedical researchers concerning growth hormone, fitness improvement, athletic performance, anti-aging, and anti–middle aging from around the world. This research has been used to design the Strategic Fitness Plans in this book.

This book is your guide to achieving new levels of health, fitness, and appearance...naturally. It begins with your commitment to following the appropriate Strategic Fitness Plan–for your age, training experience, and current fitness status–in Chapter 11 for an initial, eight-week period. Make the commitment now, but keep reading.

The Fitness Evolution

In our fast-paced world, new information impacts our lives daily. At breakneck speed, we see medicine, science, and technology moving to new levels. Medicine that was once thought to be the most advanced just a few years ago would produce malpractice claims if prescribed today.

The first comprehensive book on medicine in sports, *Hygiene des Sports,* by Sigfried Weissbein, was published in 1910. It discussed the effects of exercise on the body, injuries, and age-specific recommendations. It was not until 1979 that sports physiology and training methods—acceleration sprints, circuit training, and running intervals—were applied to sports training.

Today, major philosophies of fitness and exercise have begun to merge into a comprehensive fitness model, which is the theme of this book: increase synergistic growth hormone naturally through a comprehensive Strategic Fitness Plan based on current medical research.

The Synergy Fitness approach applies to all ages and fitness levels. The need for adults, of all ages, to improve fitness is cited by researchers. And the need crosses the full spectrum—from elite athletes to frail elderly in nursing homes, (*Training for muscular power*, 2000, Kraemer).

Fitness training is evolving toward a comprehensive fitness model that uses strategies and planning principles to get the most bang for your fitness effort. In fitness centers today, there are discussions of "cardio" after weight training. Marathoners see the value in running intervals and weight training. Bodybuilders stretch between sets and use stairmasters for cardio. And they all achieve better results.

However, there is one key component missing in most fitness plans today. And that is the need for anaerobic exercise—the sprinting, the quick-burst, out-of-breath type of running, swimming, biking, skiing, ice-skating, and hiking. The type of training should be a major player in every fitness plan because it is absolutely essential in increasing the natural release of growth hormone in your body.

Please note: If you are not a runner, do not be frightened by "sprints," or running. There are many methods (and one just right for you) of achieving the benefits of anaerobic fitness training.

You can change your appearance with this type of fitness training. Take a common sense test for a moment. The next time track and field, or Olympic swimming or speed-skating is on TV, check out the athletes in the sprinting events. Notice their physiques. Why are sprinters (of any sport) lean, muscular, cut, and so healthy in appearance?

Researchers show that the short-burst type of anaerobic exercise (like sprinting) makes your body increase GH naturally. And this book will show you how to develop a sprinter's physique—at any age.

In a study of elderly subjects (average age 79), researchers conclude that enriched food has no effect on improving the immune system. However, "exercise may prevent or slow the age-related decline in immune response." (Immunity in frail elderly: a randomized controlled trial of exercise and enriched foods, 2000, Paw).

Approximately 250,000 Americans die prematurely due to physical inactivity. (Waging war on modern chronic diseases: primary prevention through exercise biology, 2000, Booth).

Degrees of Health and Fitness

The worldwide fitness movements of weight training in the 1960s and distance running in the 1980s were effective for compulsive individuals who made time for an hour or two of training every day. However, many Americans were left behind.

Obesity in the United States is widespread and increases every year. According to a report by the Centers for Disease Control (CDC) concerning health status in America, not one state had an obesity rate above 15 percent in 1987. Four years later (while fast-food chains and channel surfing were becoming widespread), six states had reached this level, in less than 10 years. By 1998, all but six states reached this level of obesity. By 2001, the national obesity rate had reached 22 percent. What does this mean? Nearly one in four Americans are obese and 61 percent of adults are overweight. And the second most common cause of actual death is "poor diet and lack of exercise."

U.S. Surgeon General David Satcher issued a formal "Call to Action" to address the national health problems of overweight and obesity. "Overweight and obesity may soon cause as much preventable disease and death as cigarette smoking," reported Satcher.

There are 300,000 deaths a year associated with overweight and obesity, and 400,000 deaths related to tobacco. The estimated cost of these public health problems run $117 billion per year, (*Overweight and Obesity Threaten U.S. Health Gains*, December 12, 2001, HHS).

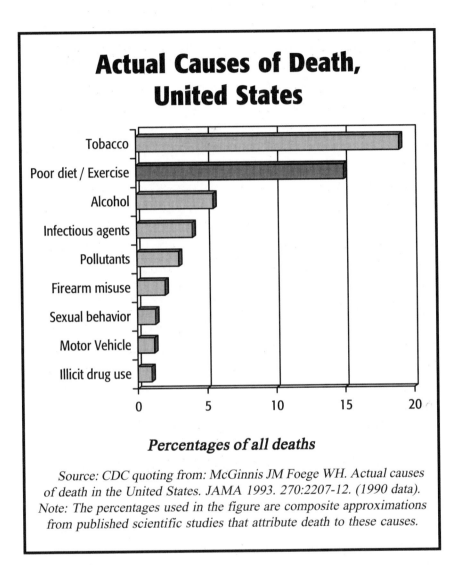

Actual Causes of Death, United States

Percentages of all deaths

Source: CDC quoting from: McGinnis JM Foege WH. Actual causes of death in the United States. JAMA 1993. 270:2207-12. (1990 data). Note: The percentages used in the figure are composite approximations from published scientific studies that attribute death to these causes.

Degrees of health and fitness are often overlooked. We are a society with two health paradigms—sick and well. Millions of Americans are one physician's visit away from being diagnosed with diabetes. Eight million Americans have undiagnosed diabetes, and 650,000 Americans will learn they have diabetes this year.

New government guidelines show that 23 million more Americans should be taking cholesterol medication to avoid a heart attack during the next 10 years, (*National Cholesterol Education Program,* 2001). And the National Institutes of Health report that 52 million Americans have cholesterol levels that exceed health recommendations. The cure: A medical prescription for exercise would be a wise national strategy.

The New Fitness Paradigm

Is there a new and better way to think about improving fitness? *Yes!* This book was written to provide you with a life changing, energy increasing, appearance improving, time-crunch efficient, fitness strategies, and a fitness plan designed for your age, and current fitness level that gets results fast.

This book also provides you with extensive fitness improvement information that is supported by medical research–not the health and fitness gimmick of the month.

From fitness newcomer to professional athlete, ***Ready, Set, GO! Synergy Fitness for Time-Crunched Adults*** offers five levels of comprehensive fitness plans designed for age, training experience, and current fitness level. Following one of the fitness plans and charting your progress in the Strategic Fitness Plan Training Log will lead you to achieve noticeable, even dramatic, improvements in fitness, appearance, and energy during the first eight weeks.

Your Strategic Fitness Plan needs to become a top priority for the next eight weeks. However, the fitness plans and the information in this book are not meant to be simply an eight week exercise blitz. This book is intended to be an exercise prescription that lasts a lifetime.

Who Needs Ready, Set, GO! Synergy Fitness for Time-Crunched Adults?

- **Middle-aged adults** wanting to lose weight, tone and build muscle, get in shape, and restore the energy levels of their youth.

- **High school, college, or professional athletes** wanting to be at peak condition for the next season.

- **Marathoners** looking to reduce time per mile and build strength in key areas for injury prevention.

- **Bodybuilders** seeking to improve symmetry by reducing body fat and adding lean fast-twitch IIa and IIx muscle fiber.

- **Physicians** writing an "exercise prescription" for their patients.

- **Adults** with diabetes or cholesterol problems.

1

Growth Hormone

Your Body's Ultimate Fat Burning, Muscle Toning and Building, Anti-aging, Anti–middle aging, Synergistic Agent

Synergy Fitness for Time-Crunched Adults is a strategically designed, comprehensive approach to fitness training with three goals:

■ Increase growth hormone (GH) in your body naturally so you can experience its many benefits (*Ready* section, Chapters 1–4).

■ Offer fully illustrated training guides that have been designed with the objective of multi-tasking exercises and major aspects of fitness training—so you can achieve maximum benefits in the shortest amount of time possible (*Set* section, Chapters 5–10).

■ Provide comprehensive, pre-designed, Strategic Fitness Plans for time-crunched adults of all ages. All in an easy-to-follow format for five Fitness Levels—based on age, current fitness status, and training experience (*GO* section, Chapter 11).

Synergy is the perfect word to describe the health and fitness impact of increasing growth hormone in your body. When growth hormone (GH) is increased, it does much more than burn calories.

Growth hormone is stored in the pituitary gland until it is "released" into the blood system. (Beyond the somatopause: growth hormone deficiency in adults over the age of 60 years, 1996, Toogood).

Growth Hormone Is Pure Fitness Synergy

Growth hormone (GH) is a natural substance produced by your body and is released in pulses—about twelve times a day. After age 18, the natural release of GH begins to decrease. And with the decrease in GH, the effects of aging begin until around age 35. At this age, what medical researchers call the "somatopause" begins.

Growth hormone is directly linked to the middle age somatopause. Its symptoms are loss of energy, fat gain (especially around the waistline), loss of bone density, and loss of lean muscle and muscle tone. Also, the skin begins to wrinkle. The great news is that medical research shows that these symptoms of aging can be delayed—even reversed.

Growth hormone creates pure fitness synergy when it is increased in your body. When growth hormone is increased naturally, through specific types of fitness training, it will tone and build muscle and stay in your body, burning fat for hours after training. And this chapter will show you how to increase growth hormone naturally, so you can enjoy the phenomenal benefits of your body's ultimate, synergistic, fitness improvement hormone.

Accidental Discovery

I discovered the type of fitness training that increases growth hormone quite by accident. I was going through middle age. And like most in the somatopause years, my metabolism was slowing, I was gaining weight around the middle (no matter what diet), and my hair was turning gray. Exercising was difficult with my work schedule. My energy level was sliding. All the signs of "middle aging" were present.

With a weight over 230 pounds (at 6′1″), and a cholesterol level of 235, I was treated for high cholesterol with the prescription drugs Lopid and Mevacor. Although I was exercising regularly, middle age was winning. Medical researchers refer to this as the somatopause. I call it the "middle age blimp-out." It describes the period when growth hormone (GH) declines to near deficient levels during the mid-30s.

I was exercising incorrectly, and could not lose weight or improve fitness. I did weight training by the circuit training method, two to three days a week at the YMCA, and I jogged for the cardio benefit three days a week. I thought it was adequate but I could not lose weight. My cardio program was by the book—achieve target heart rate and keep it there for 30 minutes. I still had high cholesterol and my weight remained at 230 pounds for several years. I tried fad diets, and (after the first few weeks of initial weight loss) I ultimately gained weight with every one. Then accidentally, I discovered growth hormone releasing exercise.

Over the years, I had played in a flag football game every Thanksgiving morning with my high school friends. We call it the Turkey Bowl. Thirty days before the game, I would usually substitute a modified sprinting-type routine for the aerobic part of my workout. During this training, I would notice muscles developing and fat dropping but I didn't catch on to the benefits of this sprinting, anaerobic exercise until after age 40.

In my early 40s, at the encouragement of Walter Diggs, Joint Commission for the Accreditation of Healthcare Organizations hospital surveyor, and Dr. Taylor Weatherby, a cardiologist friend at the hospital where I was the administrator, I entered a master's track and field competition.

My thought was that this was a health improvement goal that might help me prepare for the next Turkey Bowl. As it turned out, it did much more! It totally changed my appearance, my fitness level, and my health.

During simple anaerobic sprint training for the Turkey Bowl (which took less time than the cardio workout), I noticed my muscle increasing and my weight decreasing. Continuing the training, I also experimented with various forms of weightlifting, targeting the three types of muscle fiber and the body's three energy systems. The results were anti-aging, to say the least.

After a few months of training, I no longer needed my cholesterol drugs. My weight dropped from 230, to 220, to 210, and then to 200—without diet restriction. My body fat dropped to 10 percent. My muscles developed at youthful levels. All this with minimal changes to my diet. And today, at nearly 50, I eat. I mean, I eat...hamburgers, milkshakes, and other "not so healthy" food. As long as I follow a **Strategic Fitness Plan** in Chapter 11, I can enjoy food (in moderation of course).

The following chart shows my personal health improvements following implementation of my Strategic Fitness Plan.

Lab Reports Before and After Synergy Fitness

Lab report	Before (age 40)	After (nearly 50)	Improvement
Cholesterol	239	185	22%
Triglycerides	366	130	64%
HDL (good chol.)	29	47	62%
Weight	230	200	13%
Diet	Restrictive	Reasonable, watch excessive sugar	Enjoy meals now
Cardiac Risk	High	Zero calcification, CT cardiac profile	Significant

After training for eight weeks, I felt like I was 18 again. My energy level went sky high! And I could eat normal food and still lose weight. My fitness program worked miracles—I just didn't know why.

My running speed improved to the fastest time ever—faster even than my high school and college years. At age 45, I won a local Get-Fit Classic in the 40-yard dash event with a time of 4.69 seconds. Today, at nearly 50, I am in better shape than I was at age 20.

Others began trying my program and achieving the same remarkable results. Motivated to learn why my unique fitness plan was helping me to stay in better physical condition than 30 years earlier, I began researching to find the answer.

I read article after article about exercise and fitness but found no answers. Then one day, my wife saw an episode of the Oprah Winfrey show on anti-aging, and that led me to learn more about the miraculous anti-aging benefits of growth hormone therapy for older adults.

I began tracking medical research concerning growth hormone, and it became crystal clear—I had accidentally created a personal fitness training program that significantly increased my body's natural production of growth hormone. The results I experienced were as great as those of older adults using growth hormone replacement therapy. However, there was a huge difference—I was seeing significant results **naturally**, without hormone injections.

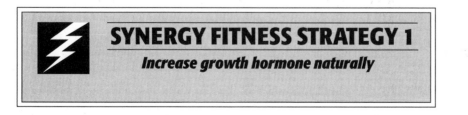

SYNERGY FITNESS STRATEGY 1

Increase growth hormone naturally

Finally, I had learned why my fitness program turned back the clock and restored my energy, reduced my weight by 30 pounds without dieting, and returned my strength, endurance, flexibility, and appearance to youthful levels.

At the encouragement of my wife, and others seeing the same great results from my fitness training plan, I decided to put my plan in writing. This turned out to be a two-year project, to share with others my Strategic Fitness Plan—with the associated medical research—for increasing growth hormone naturally.

High-Intensity Fitness Training Increases Growth Hormone Naturally

High-intensity, short-burst, sprinting type of anaerobic exercise increases growth hormone naturally. This form of training is the missing ingredient in many fitness plans today, yet it is essential in creating fitness "synergy" (getting the most benefit from your training time).

Medical research proves that anaerobic training is the best natural method to obtain the many benefits of increasing your body's supply of growth hormone. Research clearly shows that high-intensity, anaerobic fitness training—the short, hard, fast, out-of-breath, sprint type of exercise—plays a key role in increasing hormone release, *(Beta-endorphin and ACTH levels in peripheral blood during and after aerobic and anaerobic exercise,* 1986, Meirleir*).*

For athletes, increasing the intensity of training (not adding more training volume) is shown by researchers to improve athletic performance. These research findings are highlighted in Chapter 8, *Accelerating with Anaerobics,* and show that Synergy Fitness is an effective method of increasing growth hormone naturally.

"Cardio" training (aerobics) is beneficial in burning calories and providing an endurance base, and it is a key element of a well-designed fitness plan. Aerobic training is one of the five components of the Synergy Fitness. However, aerobic exercise does not have the same effect on growth hormone release as anaerobic training—and cardio takes a considerable amount of time.

The most significant recent research concerning fitness training, athletic performance improvement, anti-aging, and anti–middle aging was completed in 1999 by researchers at the University of Virginia School of Medicine. The researchers set out to determine the effects of exercise intensity on growth hormone (GH) release. They discovered that growth hormone is released in the body in direct proportion to exercise intensity—the higher the intensity, the higher the GH release, once the GH release threshold has been achieved, *(Impact of acute exercise intensity on Pulsatile growth hormone release in men,* 1999, Pritzlaff, Wideman, Weltman, Abbott, Gutgesell, Hartman, and Veldhuis). Once the research by this team becomes widely circulated, it will change the way the world thinks about exercise, fitness, health, and aging.

The state of severe oxygen deficit is called hypoxia. At high attitudes (where oxygen is thin), it is called hypoxidosis and requires treatment with oxygen therapy.

Training Intensity Increases Growth Hormone

A "particular threshold" of exercise intensity must be achieved before growth hormone is released, (*Effect of low and high intensity exercise on circulating growth hormone in men,* 1992, Felsing). This GH release threshold is determined by achieving four benchmarks during training.

You may decide to skip over the science and research concerning growth hormone (Chapters 2–4) and still achieve great results by following one of the Strategic Fitness Plans

It was once thought that the buildup of lactic acid caused muscle soreness. Not true. Lactic acid is recycled in the body before soreness appears. Soreness is caused by numerous muscle micro-tears, or overstretching the muscle during exercise. *(Delayed muscle soreness: the inflammatory response to muscle injury and its clinical implications*, 1995, MacIntyre).*

in Chapter 11. However, understanding the benchmarks that must be reached during exercise is critical to the success of your fitness plan.

Growth Hormone Release Benchmarks

Oxygen Debt

The out-of-breath condition resulting from high-intensity exercise during anaerobic training is an unmistakable GH release benchmark. This is one of those "you'll know it when you're there" destinations.

Oxygen demand and availability is an important regulator in the body's release of growth hormone during exercise, (*Regulation of growth hormone during exercise by oxygen demand and availability*, 1987, Vanhelder). Unlike other methods of fitness training, the goal of anaerobic exercise is actually to get you winded. The word *anaerobic* actually means "without oxygen."

After 6 to 8 seconds of 100 percent maximal high-intensity effort, or 8 to 30 seconds of near maximal high-intensity anaerobic exercise (like sprinting and interval training), the body goes into "oxygen debt." During recovery from this state, the body pays back the oxygen debt by increasing the heart rate and supplying oxygen to the blood with hard, rapid breathing. **It is this type of oxygen debt generated during fitness training that triggers growth hormone release.**

WARNING: Anaerobic exercise forces the heart muscle to pump fast and hard to pay back the oxygen debt caused by this form of exercise. See your physician before attempting anaerobic training.

Muscle Burn

Growth hormone release during fitness training corresponds with the "lactic acid threshold" (muscle burning sensation) that follows the "oxygen deficit" phase of high-intensity exercise.

Lactic acid (along with hydrogen ions generated during high-intensity exercise) causes a burning sensation in the muscles. Some discomfort (well, actually, a slightly painful feeling) can occur in weightlifting after 10-plus repetitions, or in running when associated with the out-of-breath condition at the end of a 100-meter sprint.

Reaching the level of "muscle burn" during fitness training is a noticeable sign that a key GH release benchmark has been reached.

Increased Body Temperature

Turn up your body heat during fitness training to increase GH. Increased body temperature is the third GH release benchmark, *(Role of body temperature in exercise-induced growth hormone and prolactin release in non-trained and physically fit subjects, 2000, Vigas).*

Note: *A good warm-up should therefore raise your body temperature by approximately one degree and this is all that's necessary for the GH release benchmark.*

Even in outdoor temperatures reaching freezing, body heat can be raised with adequate clothing. So do not let cold weather be an excuse. There are temperatures, however, that will preclude GH from being released. Working up a good "sweat" during training should accomplish this GH release benchmark!

> *Researchers demonstrate that GH will not release when exercise occurs in a cold room where body temperature cannot increase.* (Characterization of growth hormone release in response to external heating: Comparison to exercise induced release, 1984 Christensen).

The increase of GH during exercise is closely correlated with the release of adrenal hormones (adrenaline and norepinephrine). This occurs after reaching the "lactate threshold" benchmark.

(Threshold increases in plasma growth hormone in relation to plasma catecholamine and blood lactate concentration during progressive exercise in endurance-training athletes, 1996, Chwalbinski-Moneta).

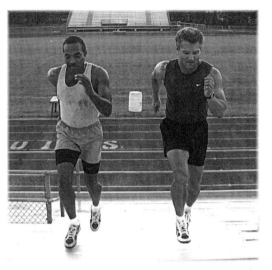

Running bleachers will achieve GH release benchmarks.

Adrenal Response

The University of Virginia research team identified the "adrenal (kidney) hormone release function" as possibly playing the central role in GH release. The release of epinephrine (adrenaline) that boosts the body in stressful situations and norepinephrine, which maintains normal blood circulation, both play vital roles in GH release. So fitness training must achieve the out-of-breath, slightly painful level of intensity that produces an epinephrine (adrenaline) response before GH is released.

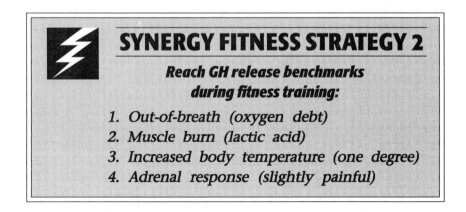

SYNERGY FITNESS STRATEGY 2

Reach GH release benchmarks during fitness training:

1. *Out-of-breath (oxygen debt)*
2. *Muscle burn (lactic acid)*
3. *Increased body temperature (one degree)*
4. *Adrenal response (slightly painful)*

It is not age, but the intensity of training that determines the success of this GH release benchmark. In one study, young and old adults were tested for their ability to release norepinephrine during exercise. There was no statistical difference in performance at any age, (*Young and old subjects matched for aerobic capacity have similar noradrenergic responses to exercise*, 1993, Kastello).

GH release occurs 16 minutes after reaching the muscle burn lactate threshold benchmark during exercise. (Growth hormone responses during intermittent weightlifting exercise in men, 1984, Vanhelder).

Timing of GH Release Following Exercise

The timing of GH release after exercise has been measured to the "muscle burn" lactate production in the body because lactate (a GH release benchmark) is a standard measurement for exercise physiologists. However, lactate has been proven *not* to be the exclusive cause for GH release, (Lugar, 1992). Lactic acid increases during training and occurs almost simultaneously with the out-of-breath, muscle-burning, slightly painful (adrenal response) type of high intensity exercise, (Weltman, 1997).

Growth hormone increases "significantly" at the end of 20 minutes of 85 percent intensity exercise. GH peaks approximately one hour into the recovery period. And GH levels return to baseline two to three hours after training, (*Effects of blood pH and blood lactate on growth hormone, prolactin, and gonadotropin release after acute exercise in male volunteers*, 1997, Slias).

This means that after you reach GH release benchmarks during training, GH will remain in your system burning fat for two to three hours during recovery. You create a powerful fat burning system—*naturally*—once you achieve growth hormone release during exercise. This is "fitness synergy!"

Want GH Synergistically Burning Fat for Hours After Training?

Implement these three strategies before, during and after your workouts. Avoid high fat meals for one hour before training. During training, drink lots of water. Avoid high sugar foods (dessert, candy, **sugar drinks**) after your workout for two to three hours. And take 25 grams of protein after training.

1. BEFORE Training GH Strategy:
No High Fat Meals One Hour Before Training

A high fat meal before training stops growth hormone cold, according to researchers, (*Acute effects of high fat and high glucose meals on the growth hormone response to exercise*, 1993, Cappon).

High fat meals trigger an increase in a hormone called somatostatin, which inhibits growth hormone. It is important to limit any activity that increases somatostatin because of its negative impact on GH. So to get the most from a workout, no high fat meals one hour before training.

2. DURING Training GH Strategy:
Drink Lots of Water

Inadequate fluid during training hurts exercise-induced GH release. Research in 2001 shows that inadequate water intake during fitness training will "significantly" reduce the GH response to fitness training, (*Effect of hydration on exercise-induced growth hormone response*, 2001, Peyreigne).

AFTER Training GH Strategy:
No Sugar for Two Hours

A high sugar meal, or even a recovery drink (containing high sugar) after training, may stop the benefits of growth hormone generated during your training. You can work out for hours, but eat a high sugar candy bar, or high sugar energy drink and you will shut down the synergistic benefits of GH.

Even before training, a high sugar meal will slightly impair GH, but after training, consider your exercise induced growth hormone release stopped.

Growth hormone in your system stimulates fat burning during the two to three hour recovery period after training. If you do not reach GH release during training (due to lack of intensity), you will still achieve the calorie burning benefit from the workout. However, you will miss the growth hormone "synergy bonus" of fat burning for two to three hours after training.

This is an extremely important fact if you want to shed a few pounds. You can lose fat dramatically by increasing GH during training and not eating refined sugar.

The University of Virginia research demonstrates that carbohydrates are burned during exercise in direct proportion to the intensity of training. And fat burning is correlated with intensity. However, fat burning takes place *after* the workout, during the recovery period.

Researchers find that protein supplements improve muscle protein balance for middle age and elderly adults who use resistance training in their fitness plan. (The utility of resistance exercise training and amino acid supplementation for reversing age-associated decrements in muscle protein mass and function, 2000, Parise).

The Ultimate Fat Burning Synergistic Agent

Since the increase in GH that burns fat after training lasts for two or more hours, **when GH is released during a workout, your body continues to burn fat for two or more hours afterwards.** You get much more than just the calories burned during fitness training when you release GH.

Keep in mind, normal aerobic exercise and typical fitness programs will not achieve GH release benchmarks.

It takes a strategically designed fitness plan (like the plans prescribed in Chapter 11) that includes anaerobic training as a major focus to accomplish GH release.

AFTER Training Strategy: 25 Grams of Protein

While high fat meals before training and sugar afterwards limit growth hormone, researchers have found that protein after training is beneficial, (*Acute amino acids supplementation enhances pituitary responsiveness in athletes*, Di Luigi, 1999). After training, amino acid transport (protein utilization) increases during the recovery period, (Bilol, 1995). A protein supplement (without concentrated sugar) or a high protein meal with 25 grams of protein after fitness training is a wise muscle toning and building, and body fat reducing strategy.

Protein supplements sold in large canisters with two scoops totaling approximately 25 to 50 grams are a convenient source of protein—except one scoop of 25 grams is sufficient for most individuals.

The 25 Gram Protein List

Protein Supplement	1 scoop
Chicken / Fish / Beef	4 oz.
Nutritional Yeast	8 tbs.
Beef/Turkey Jerky	1 cup
Water-packed Tuna	6 oz.
Eggs	3

Specific details for high-intensity training protein needs can be found in a chart on page 58, *"Daily Protein Needs."* You can also find the latest research information concerning protein requirements for high-intensity fitness training on the Web at www.readysetgofitness.com

Conclusion

To receive the synergistic benefits of growth hormone, you must reach all four GH release benchmarks during training.

- Perform anaerobic high-intensity, out-of-breath exercise.
- Raise body temperature during fitness training.
- Reach muscle burn (lactic acid) while training.
- Achieve slightly painful adrenal response though high-intensity exercise.

After reaching growth hormone release benchmarks during fitness training, growth hormone will peak and remain in your body for two to three hours burning fat. To maximize this fat burning synergy bonus, implement the following strategies:

BEFORE training: No high fat meals for one hour.

DURING training: Drink lots of water.

AFTER training: No sugar for two hours.

                    Intake 25 grams of protein.

The next chapter, *Rediscovering the Energy of Your Youth*, will cover essential information about growth hormone medical research.

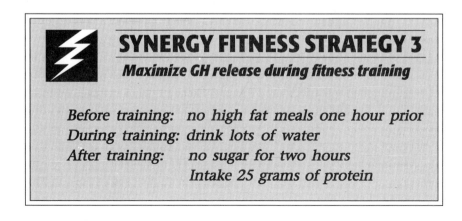

SYNERGY FITNESS STRATEGY 3
Maximize GH release during fitness training

Before training: no high fat meals one hour prior
During training: drink lots of water
After training: no sugar for two hours
                   Intake 25 grams of protein

2

Rediscovering the Energy of Your Youth

The key to rediscovering the energy of your youth is increasing growth hormone (GH) to youthful levels. The key to optimum health, fitness, and athletic performance, is, you got it: increasing your body's natural release of growth hormone.

"But doesn't growth hormone make you grow?" This is a frequent question. Growth hormone does not make adults grow taller or bigger. It burns fat, increases bone density, tones and builds muscles, and improves skin and appearance.

Whether you are a high school athlete wishing to improve your athletic performance, middle-aged and wanting to get into shape, or maybe a senior citizen who has read about the anti-aging research demonstrating that growth hormone treatments can reverse the effects of aging by 20 years—step one is learning about growth hormone. Let me go one more step. Actually, you need to become a near-expert concerning the activities that increase the release of this hormone in order to best utilize it in your own body.

Professional athlete or great-grandmother, increasing growth hormone *naturally* should become your top fitness goal. And step one is learning how growth hormone functions in your body.

Obviously, all hormones produced by the body are important. However, the way you stimulate the release of GH naturally—through diet, nutritional supplements, sleep, and GH-releasing exercise—will typically determine the functional outcome of other hormones. In other words, if your fitness and nutrition plans are on target with growth hormone, the other hormones in your body will typically be well managed.

Growth hormone may do more than you ever imagined. This hormone impacts every aspect of life, for your entire lifetime. GH affects your career, appearance, self-image, ambition, energy, and performance—both physical and mental. Even relationships with family and friends are affected by growth hormone.

Understanding how growth hormone functions will impact the way you think about fitness training—and may lead you to modify your diet, add specific nutritional supplements, and perhaps even change your sleeping patterns. Understanding how specific types of fitness training impact the body's natural release of GH will cause you to rethink current methods of fitness training.

Why Is Growth Hormone So Hot?

Growth hormone is extremely popular with elite athletes, bodybuilders, entertainment celebrities, and patients at anti-aging centers seeking age-reversing therapies.

Filmmaker Oliver Stone, actor Nick Nolte, and actress Dixie Carter all acknowledge using GH, according to Ann Oldenburg of *USA Today* (November 14, 2000). She quotes Ken Dychtwall of Age Wave, who estimates that there are 250,000 Americans injecting GH. Even at a cost of $12,000 a year, it's clear that GH is popular.

At the 2000 summer Olympics in Sydney, Australia, there was a global focus placed on GH due to suspected abuse of performance-enhancing drugs. GH is currently undetectable as an illegal athletic performance improvement substance.

Now that GH has made the rounds in Hollywood and international athletic circles, it could move mainstream. Unfortunately, in the not too distant future, we may read that high school athletes are using GH injections to enhance performance, lose weight, and improve appearance.

While reading about the many benefits of increasing GH in this chapter, you will learn about GH injections. However, GH injections are not recommended unless your lab report states "GH deficient" and you have discussed the risks with your physician.

Injecting growth hormone does add additional GH to the system. Unfortunately, this triggers the body to suppress its *own* production of GH. It's true that higher GH levels will produce wonderful benefits through injections. However, there is a better, safer way.

The purpose of this book is to show you how to increase this youth-rejuvenating, athletic performance enhancing hormone, *naturally,* through a strategic fitness plan, balanced diet, nutritional supplements, and "slow wave" deep sleep.

Side Effects of GH Injections

Side effects of GH injections in healthy individuals can be serious. They include acromegaly, a condition that causes short bones in the face, hands, and feet to grow unusually large. This condition leaves the individual with a "Neanderthal" appearance. And it is permanent—there is no cure. However, increasing GH naturally has been shown not to cause this condition.

Also, research on lab mice shows an increase of liver tumors with GH. Basically, when the mouse has a tumor, GH appears to enhance its growth, (*Overexpressed growth hormone [GH] synergistically promotes carcinogen-initiated liver tumor growth by promoting cellular proliferation in emerging hepatocellular neoplasms in female and male GH-transgenic mice, 2001, Snibson*). Clearly, natural methods are the optimum way to receive the benefits of growth hormone.

Role of Growth Hormone

GH is one of over a hundred hormones released naturally in the body. Hormones are often described as the body's "messengers," because they are chemicals that transfer information and instructions between cells. GH is released by the pituitary gland, often called the "master gland," which secretes several important hormones as well. These hormones regulate metabolism; control the body's water balance; and manage secretions of estrogen and progesterone and the creation of testosterone—the essential hormone in muscle development and sex drive. The pituitary gland also controls the release of endorphins—the body's natural pain relievers.

GH is a powerful hormone responsible for promoting and regulating muscle and tissue growth, regulating carbohydrate and fat metabolism, and controlling other vital glands.

Functions of Growth Hormone:

· Dictates growth rates in children
· Controls "rapid growth spurt" in adolescents
· Increases protein metabolism to build muscle
· Breaks down lipids (fats)
· Increases retention of vital minerals
· Enhances cartilage growth and bone formation
· Decreases bad LDL cholesterol
· Increases good HDL cholesterol
· Stimulates release of other essential hormones

"The Methuselah factor is contained within the pituitary system."

James Jamieson, pharmacologist and author, *Growth Hormone: Reversing the Aging Process Naturally. The Methuselah Factor,* 1997).

Methuselah was the longest living human in recorded history.

Growth hormone keeps your body youthful in appearance. In fact, GH could be described as the "appearance hormone."

Growth Hormone Declines with Age, Unless...

Growth hormone declines with age, unless you implement a strategy to increase it. And that strategy should include a fitness plan targeted at increasing GH release during training.

GH declines at a rate of 14 percent every decade. By age 40, GH has typically dropped by 50 percent from youthful levels. By age 55, GH will drop 80 percent unless a strategy to increase GH release is implemented. The following graph shows the drastic decline of GH from age 14 to age 25.

Growth Hormone Declines with Age

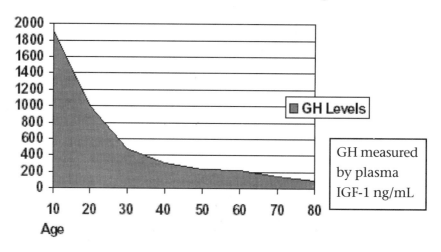

The mental image of GH release during the life cycle is one of 10-year-old children running, jumping, sprinting, and playing, with GH surging through their bodies to provide significant growth in height until the late teens, at which point GH begins to decline.

By the mid-30s, the decline of growth hormone reaches a threshold level. And this level triggers what medical researchers refer to as the "somatopause," the metabolism slow-down, waist/hips expansion, weight gain period of middle age.

Characteristics of somatopause include gray hair, decrease in energy, decrease in lean muscle, increase in body fat (especially around the middle), cardiovascular disease, decrease in sex drive, osteoporosis, facial wrinkles, and other signs of middle-aging as we know it. When you hear a 35-year-old say, "my metabolism is slowing down" or "I can't keep the weight off" he or she is describing somatopause.

Can the Effects of Somatopause be Delayed?

The answer is **yes!**

In older adults, when GH is returned to youthful levels through GH injections, the reports are near miraculous—increases in energy, sex drive, lean muscle, and bone density, and decreases in body fat, even some reports of gray hair returning to youthful colors...no kidding! And these reports are based on scientific medical research conducted by physicians.

Are GH injections the fountain of youth? No, but increasing GH through **natural** means may be as close as we can come. Let us look more closely at GH research. Don't tune out. This brief history lesson will not be too painful.

Growth Hormone Medical History

Dr. Harvey Cushing officially discovered growth hormone in 1912. He named it "the hormone of growth." Little happened until 1956, when Dr. Maurice Raben isolated GH from human cadavers and injected it in 1958 into a dwarf child. Miraculously, the child began to grow taller.

The time and effort involved in extracting GH from human cadavers and animals—and a dose of mad cow disease in an early batch—slowed the use of GH. The FDA approved synthetic (man-made) GH in 1985. Protropin was the name given by Genentech for synthetic GH, and it was exclusively used to treat dwarfism in children.

The annual cost of treatment is $12,000 per child. Today, 30,000 children are growing normally, due to the work of medical researchers. GH injections for children with dwarfism are miraculous. Just talk to a parent of a child suffering from this condition, now growing as any other child.

Growth Hormone Becomes Famous

Doctors seeking the answer to one question made growth hormone famous. *Since synthetic GH injections restore near normal growth in GH-deficient children, would increasing GH to youthful levels in older adults reverse the effects of aging?*

Dr. Daniel Rudman and colleagues conducted an experiment to answer this question. Their findings changed the course of medical research. In one of the most famous experiments in modern medicine, 12 healthy men—ages 61 to 80—were injected with synthetic GH three times a week for six months. The results were incredible. The injections restored GH-deficient levels (less than 350 units per liter measured by IGF-1 in blood serum) to youthful levels (500 to 1500) and subsequently **reversed the effects of several years of aging.**

An important point—the adults were instructed not to change their lifestyles in any way so that the impact of GH would be isolated during the study. The men gained 8.8 percent muscle mass, lost 14.4 percent body fat, and made age-reversing improvements in bone density and skin thickness.

Dr. Rudman and colleagues published their research findings in the *New England Journal of Medicine* July 5 ,1990. The article, *Effects of human growth hormone in men over 60 years old,* The researchers concluded:

> *"The findings in this study are consistent with the hypothesis that the decrease in lean body mass, the increase in adipose-tissue mass, and the thinning of the skin that occur in older men are caused in part by reduced activity of the growth hormone—IGF-1 axis, and can be restored in part by the administration of human growth hormone. The effects of six months of human growth hormone on lean body mass, adipose tissue mass, were equivalent in magnitude to the changes incurred during ten to twenty years of aging."*

The effects of increasing human growth hormone for six months were equivalent in magnitude to the changes incurred during 10 to 20 years of aging.

GH reverses hardening of the arteries, and if maintained, GH treatment reduces morbidity and mortality rates in GH deficient adults. (Growth hormone treatment reverses early atherosclerotic changes in GH-deficient adults, 1999, Pfeifer).

Dr. Edmund Chein, director, and Dr. Vogt of the Palm Springs Life Extension Institute and Dr. Terry of the Medical College of Wisconsin conducted experiments with 2,000 adults from 1994 to 1998 using low dose and high frequency of self administered GH injections. Their results in round numbers: 10 percent increase in lean muscle (this would make any bodybuilder proud) and 10 percent decrease in body fat after six months of treatment. Dr. Chein and colleagues support a comprehensive approach of resistance training, endurance exercises, appropriate nutrition, and stress reduction with GH replacement therapy. For readers who are clearly GH-deficient and are considering GH replacement therapy, Dr. Chein has an informative Website at www.drchein.com.

Cutting-Edge Growth Hormone Research

New medical research taking place with GH treatment is exciting, so exciting that the Growth Hormone Research Society has been formed. Reported medical outcomes of GH research are typically positive and call for additional study into new unexplored areas.

Only one main negative has emerged thus far, and it deals with GH treatment of critically ill patients. Researchers report that GH for critically ill patients actually increases mortality, prolongs ventilation, and increases the number of hospital intensive care days, (*Increased mortality associated with growth hormone treatment in critically ill adults*, 1999, Takala). Therefore, it seems that GH treatment does not have value in a hospital critical care unit. But as a health preventative, youth rejuvenating, fitness improving stimulant, GH has demonstrated positive outcomes.

Under new medical definitions, most middle-aged adults are GH deficient—particularly those who are overweight and do not exercise to stimulate GH release. A total fitness program may not only change your appearance and improve fitness, a well-planned fitness program may extend your life by decreasing your risk of vascular disease.

A total fitness program may not only change your appearance and improve fitness, a well-planned fitness program may extend your life by decreasing your risk of vascular disease.

During one of the longest research studies on growth hormone (10 years), researchers report:

"Ten year GH therapy in adults with GH-D (GH-Deficiency) increases lean body and muscle mass, decreases carotid intima media thickness, and produces a less atherogenic lipid profile," (GH lowers cholesterol).

Additional significant findings in this report are increases in energy levels and decreases in LDL cholesterol (bad cholesterol). GH therapy also improves psychological well-being, researchers report:

"The Nottingham Health Profile, used to assess psychological well-being, showed improvement in overall scores, energy levels, and emotional reaction in the GH-treated patients compared with the untreated patients," (*The effects of 10 years of recombinant growth hormone (GH) in adult GH-deficient patients*, 1999, Gibney).

GH has stirred a great interest in the medical research community. Results of GH treatment are typically positive, and have far reaching implications.

Are GH injections the fountain of youth? As stated earlier, no. However, increasing GH through diet, nutritional supplements, appropriate "slow wave" deep sleep, and, most importantly, consistently following a GH-increasing Strategic Fitness Plan in this book, may be as close as anything discovered to date.

Growth Hormone Released in Pulses

The pituitary gland manufactures GH. The pea-size pituitary gland is located at the base of the brain about one inch behind your nose. In normal individuals, the pituitary manufactures 0.4 mg to 1.0 mg of GH per day and stores 5 to 10 mg. Individuals using high intensity exercise—like the Strategic Fitness Plans in this book—manufacture and store even higher levels of GH.

The hypothalamus gland (located just above the pituitary) controls the number of GH pulses, and the amount of GH released in each pulse...

I know what you're thinking—Wait just a minute, this is getting complicated. And you're right! However, understanding the basics of GH release is vitally important to the success of your fitness program.

The hypothalamus gland, located deep within the brain just behind the eyes, is connected with the pituitary gland by nerve endings. It is the connecting link between the brain and the pituitary, receiving messages from the brain and sending instructions to the pituitary through hormones. Then the pituitary does the work.

GH is not released into the body in a consistent supply to the blood stream. GH is released in pulses. During youth, there are typically 12 daily pulses of GH. As we age, the number of pulses decline, and the amount of GH released during the pulses also decreases. (1990, Wideman).

In a thermostat-type regulating method, there are two hormones that control GH release. The two hormones released by the hypothalamus to control GH release are growth hormone releasing hormone (GHRH) and somatostatin. GHRH stimulates the pituitary to release GH. Somatostatin inhibits GH release.

Your goal should be to increase GHRH without releasing somatostatin, using a two-pronged strategy. Simply, do things to increase GHRH, and do not do things to release somatostatin.

Stress Increases Somatostatin and Stops GH Release

Stress causes many physical reactions in the body. One of these is an increase in somatostatin. In an experiment, researchers administered anti-serums to stop somatostatin release in rats just prior to the onset of stress. The anti-serums somewhat restored the growth hormone that had been essentially stopped by stress.

Although, the subjects of this study were rats and not humans, it can be safely concluded that high stress will stop growth hormone release, due to excessive levels of somatostatin, *(Antiserum to somatostatin prevents stress-induced inhibition of growth hormone in the rat, 1976, Terry)*.

Fitness training can often help individuals cope with stress. Depending on individual situations, stress reduction may take more than exercise, but the important point is to know that stress will inhibit growth hormone release, and you can do something about it.

Conclusion

Growth hormone release is vitally important in achieving optimum health, fitness and appearance at any age. Middle age and older adults may receive the most benefits from increasing GH naturally.

Methods of increasing GH that apply to a high school athlete also apply to the athlete's mom and dad, and even their grandmother and grandfather. The following chapter discusses five strategies to increase growth hormone in your body.

It was not until the 1970s that we learned how the pituitary controlled GH. Drs. Roger Guilleman, Andrew Schalyl and Rosalyn Yalow received the Nobel prize in 1977 for discovering how GHRH (+) and somatostatin (-) regulate the release of GH.

3

How to Improve Athletic Performance, Delay the Middle Age Somatopause, and Reverse Effects of Aging by 20 Years

Growth hormone plays a vital role in improving fitness, athletic performance, anti-aging, and anti–middle aging efforts. No matter what your age or fitness condition, increasing growth hormone (GH) naturally should become your top fitness training goal.

In describing ways to increase GH in your body, I use the description "GH release." GH is stored in the pituitary until it's "released" into the blood system. This occurs naturally when certain thresholds are reached with diet, sleep, and exercise.

Natural GH Release Strategies

- **Adequate "slow wave" sleep**
- **GH enhancing nutritional supplements**
- **GH secretagogues**
- **GH releasing exercise**

While GH replacement therapy by injection is an appropriate treatment in certain situations, this is not natural and should be a "last resort," reserved for GH-deficient individuals. No borderline decisions here. The lab report must clearly register "GH deficient." And this decision should involve discussions with your trusted primary care provider, family medicine physician, internist, or OB-GYN.

GH injections take the place of the body's own natural GH secretions, whereas specific types of fitness training (Chapters 5–11) will increase GH naturally, without injections.

GH secretagogues (sa-KREE-ta-gogs) and GH-enhancing nutritional supplements are similar, yet different. Some experts may argue with my definition because, theoretically, nutritional supplements that increase GH secretion would be considered GH secretagogues. But supplements are usually formed from a single amino acid while powerful GH secretagogues are a complex mixture of several amino acids.

GH secretagogues can actually range from potent compounds of several amino acids and other protein transport agents to prescription medications. GH enhancing supplements are available over-the-counter at most nutrition stores. True, some GH secretagogues can be derived naturally and rightfully wear the title of "natural."

For the purpose of understanding GH-releasing strategies, however, a distinction must be made between "L-glutamine" an amino acid supplement and the secretagogue "symbiotropin," for example.

GH secretagogues may be a backup strategy if natural methods are not effective. It is wise to first give a full effort to GH-producing exercise and nutritional supplements. However, if you do not obtain reasonable results from this strategy and want to consider GH secretagogues, I recommend reading James Jamieson's book, *Growth Hormone: Reversing Human Aging Naturally*, (*Longevity News Network*, 1997). And of course, discuss this strategy thoroughly with your physician.

However, increasing your body's *natural* GH release through exercise is hopefully why you purchased this book. Current medical research is crystal clear—exercise has a profound effect on GH release, (*Growth Hormone and Exercise*, 1999, Jenkins).

Research at the University of Virginia demonstrates that exercise increases the frequency of GH releases and the amount of GH released per pulse/secretion in a linear relationship to the intensity of exercise. (Impact of acute exercise intensity on pulsatile growth hormone release in men, 1999, Pritzlaff).

Adopt the Synergy Fitness Strategy of Increasing GH Naturally by:

(1) Commit to following a Strategic Fitness Plan—suited for your age, training experience, and current fitness level for an initial eight-week period.

(2) Follow a GH-release enhancing diet—balanced diet in moderation, high protein, low refined sugar, adequate carbs and fat, and nutritional supplements--proven by research to stimulate GH release.

(3) Get adequate "slow wave" deep sleep.

Melatonin supplements have been successful in treating sleep problems for shift work, jet lag, and some sleep disorders.
(Melatonin II: physiological and therapeutic effects, 2000, Bruls).

GH Released During "Slow Wave" Sleep

The largest release of GH occurs during the first phases of "slow wave" deep sleep, about two hours into sleep, (*Thirty-second sampling of plasma growth hormone in man: correlation with sleep stages,* 1991, Holl).

As we age, our sleep quality decreases, and so does the nighttime release of GH. This decrease in GH runs "directly parallel" to the decrease in slow wave sleep, (*Age-related changes in slow wave sleep and REM sleep and relationship with growth hormone and cortisol levels in healthy men,* 2000, Van Cauter). Adequate sleep is a critical GH-release strategy. In a similar study, researchers even suggest that there may be a future role for medicine to assist the nighttime release of GH during slow wave sleep, (*Interrelationships between growth hormone and sleep,* 2000, Van Cauter).

Melatonin Supplements Aid Sleep

Melatonin is a hormone that is made from eating protein, specifically the amino acid tryptophan, and it is the most powerful regulator of the body's biological clock. Melatonin increases at night and decreases during the day in a light-dark cycle. During childhood, melatonin is released in higher levels, resulting in more slow wave deep sleep.

Melatonin supplements are inexpensive, widely used, and seemingly effective as sleep aids. In one year, 20 million Americans purchased melatonin supplements to self-treat their sleep problems. Some medical researchers feel that melatonin supplements are abused and have called for additional investigation concerning self-treatment of sleep disorders with this supplement, (*Melatonin: aeromedical, toxicopharmaclological, and analytical,* 1999, Sanders).

While melatonin seems to be an effective supplement, there are unanswered questions. Personally, I have tried melatonin supplements. They do make me sleep; however, I am sluggish the next day, and because of that I do not like using them. Using melatonin for jet lag, for a night or two a year when needed, seems reasonable. Some bodybuilders take melatonin supplements nightly in the hope of increasing their nighttime release of GH. Excessive? Probably, because the research is not conclusive.

How important is the GH release during sleep? Researchers report that patients with chronic fatigue syndrome/fibromyalgia have significantly lower night secretion levels of GH. Current research cannot determine if low nocturnal GH secretion is the cause or an effect of these conditions, (Berwaerts, 1998). Clinical trials are being conducted at a major university to study the impact of GH injections on adults with chronic fatigue syndrome.

Dark conditions increase the natural increase of melatonin at night. Since adequate slow wave sleep is an important GH release strategy, dark sleeping conditions may promote GH release during sleep. (Secretion of growth hormone in patients with chronic fatigue, 1998, Berwaerts).

Protein During the Day
Aids Sleep at Night

A balanced diet with adequate protein during the day will help you achieve quality sleep, and in turn assist GH release at night. Most protein-rich foods (meat, chicken, fish) contain the amino acid tryptophan, which produces melatonin for sleep. Adequate protein intake during the day will allow your body to build up plenty of melatonin for natural sleep at night.

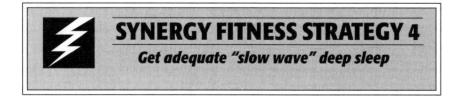

SYNERGY FITNESS STRATEGY 4
Get adequate "slow wave" deep sleep

DAILY PROTEIN NEEDS

FOR MEDIUM-INTENSITY AND HIGH-INTENSITY FITNESS PROGRAMS

Weight	Medium-Intensity Training*	High-Intensity Training**
100 lbs.	60–75 grams	100–120 grams
150 lbs.	90–112 grams	150–180 grams
200 lbs.	120–150 grams	200–240 grams

*Medium-Intensity formula: 0.6 to 0.75 grams of protein per lb. bodyweight.
**High-Intensity formula: 1 to 1.2 grams per lb. bodyweight.

Twenty-two amino acids make up protein, the body's building blocks for growth and maintenance. Eleven amino acids are produced by the body itself, and the other amino acids are classified as essential, meaning they must come from the diet.

GH Release Enhancing Nutritional Supplements

Medical research about increasing growth hormone through nutritional supplements is rapidly advancing but far from complete. Studies have targeted protein and the current thinking is that inexpensive nutritional supplements composed of single amino acids increase growth hormone.

Specific amino acid supplements are successful in increasing the release of growth hormone naturally by blocking GH inhibitors and stimulating GH release.

Glutamine
World Champion GH Supplement

L-glutamine is an inexpensive, single amino acid supplement that has been shown by researchers to be effective in increasing growth hormone. Glutamine also has a positive immune system function. Henry Mallek, author of *The Longevity Diet*, states:

> *The idea is to think nutrients. Instead of telling you to eat beans for protein, Mallek says, "think glutamine." That's because the principle anti-aging benefit of glutamine, found in beans, maintains a supply of antioxidants in the body.*

(*USA Today*, November 14, 2000)

In *Growth Hormone: Reversing Human Aging Naturally*, author and pharmacologist James Jamieson cites research showing a 15 percent increase in GH from glutamine supplementation. Jamieson's book provides an excellent survey of medical research regarding growth hormone and an effective viewpoint of increasing GH from a secretagogue release strategy.

A dose of 2 grams of glutamine (typically two 1000 mg tablets) on an empty stomach with a carbonated drink will increase GH release. Why carbonation? Jamieson theorizes that carbonation provides necessary "chaperone molecules," ensuring that the glutamine gets to the right GH pituitary receptors. Another report states that water is better than carbonation. However, the "chaperone theory" seems to have support in the literature. Hopefully, forthcoming research will clarify this question.

High-intensity fitness training can drop normal glutamine levels in the blood system by as much as 50 percent. This makes glutamine supplementation possibly a wise pre-training strategy.

A noteworthy research study at Louisiana State University shows that growth hormone increases significantly 90 minutes after taking 2 grams of glutamine dissolved in cola. (Increased plasma bicarbonate and growth hormone after an oral glutamine load, 1995, Welbourne).

The American College of Sports Medicine reports that masters athletes (over age 30) have elevated nutritional needs over younger athletes. (Masters athletes: factors affecting performance, 1999, Marharam).

However, while the research is close, it is not yet conclusive. I take 2 grams of glutamine prior to training, and it seems to have a positive effect at the end of my workout. Glutamine does not produce a temperature-increasing "thermogenic boost" (like caffeine from a cup of coffee, or the ephedrine boost from the herbs ma hung and guarana). At the end of a workout, I feel like I have extra stamina, and this allows me to train with more intensity at the end of the workout. Many readers have told me they also get the same effect from 2 grams of glutamine before training.

In one study, researchers report that after completion of a marathon, blood glutamine levels drop significantly, (*Some aspects of the acute phase response after a marathon race, and the effects of glutamine supplementation*, 1997, Castell). The fact that many athletes experience colds following a marathon leads one to wonder if the drastic drop in blood glutamine plays a role in causing the colds. Would glutamine supplementation before training and before the marathon help avoid them?

"Overtraining just prior to competition" is the standard reason given for the illness-after-the-event phenomenon, but Castell's conclusion regarding the glutamine drop caused by the marathon appears to be reasonable. Clearly, those who participate in high-intensity fitness training need to replenish nutrients used to generate energy during athletic competitions and training. Therefore, it may be a reasonable fitness strategy to consider supplementing with 2 grams of glutamine prior to training.

Pre-workout glutamine supplementation has also been shown by researchers to reduce the post-exercise decline in blood glutamine levels, (*Effects of glutamine supplementation on exercise-induced changes in lymphocyte function*, 2001, Krzywkowski).

Initial research seems to show that glutamine supplementation before training may be a wise fitness strategy. More research is necessary to clarify the exact role and potential side effects of glutamine. The Synergy Fitness Website www.readysetgofitness.com will track research concerning the role of glutamine as a possible pre-training strategy.

Somatostatin is the hormone that acts in opposition to the positive GH release in a thermostat type regulating function. (1996, Calabresi).

Glutamine has drug interactions with the chemotherapy drugs Taxol and Paclitaxel. Ask your doctor or pharmacist if you have questions. GNC has an informative section on their Website for checking drug interactions with nutrition supplements (www.gnc.com). And the National Library of Medicine has an excellent Website at www.medlineplus.gov, click on the "Drug Information" link. This site has over 11 million citations from worldwide medical journals and is visited over 28 million times a month.

Arginine

The effect of L-arginine (amino acid) on the release of GH was recently studied at the University of Virginia. Researchers concluded that arginine assists the positive GH-releasing effect of exercise by limiting somatostatin release, (*Synergy of L-Arginine and GHRP-2 stimulation of growth hormone in men and women: modulation by exercise,* 2000, Wideman).

One study successfully used 1.5 grams of arginine to increase the impact of GH release by blocking somatostatin. Some experts suggest taking arginine and glutamine on an empty stomach after a workout and before bed to further increase GH release.

Large amounts of arginine have been used successfully with another amino acid, ornithine, to increase GH release. Ornithine is manufactured in the body when arginine is used during the production of urea. The literature suggests that these two amino acids may promote muscle building by increasing GH and insulin. However, the amount of arginine used in the study, 13 grams, caused gastrointestinal problems.

The bottom line on arginine as a viable GH release agent is far from complete. One study from UCLA shows that arginine produces no increase in GH with exercise and actually may impair GH release during weight training, (Oral *arginine does not stimulate basal or augment exercise-induced GH secretion in either young or old adults*, 1999, Marcell).

Arginine can inflame cold sores. Arginine has no known drug interactions published at this time. However, adults using lysine for the treatment of cold sores (inflamed by stress and sun exposure) may not want to use arginine during the treatment phase because arginine can stimulate the virus that causes cold sores. For this reason and conflicting research studies, I do not take arginine as an individual supplement.

Arginine does have one noteworthy side effect. It produces nitric oxide, a key amino acid used in herbal formula Viagra alternatives. You may want to keep this in mind the next time an herbal potency ad comes on TV—you may already have a key ingredient on your vitamin shelf.

Lysine

L-lysine is an essential amino acid and is most famous for treating cold sores by interfering with the herpes simplex virus. By incorporating itself into many proteins, lysine acts as a partner with other amino acids, particularly those involving nitrogen metabolism, calcium absorption, and promotion of growth and lean body mass.

Due to the partnering role of lysine with other amino acids, it is frequently used in nutritional "stacks" —combinations of various amino acids, vitamins, and herbs to create compounds.

Researchers at the University of Houston demonstrate that 1,500 milligrams of lysine and 1,500 milligrams of arginine immediately before exercise does not change exercise-induced GH. These supplements do, however, increase GH under normal, non-exercising activity. Arginine supplements, then, may be better utilized when taken several hours prior to or following exercise, (*Acute effect of amino acid ingestion and resistance exercise on plasma growth hormone concentration in young men*, Sumunski, 1997).

> *Researchers report that the current World Health Organization recommendation concerning lysine should be three times higher.* (Dietary lysine requirement of young adult males determined by oxidation of L-[1-13C] phenylalanine, 1993, Zello).

Niacin

Niacin (vitamin B-3) enhances GH release by reducing fatty acids. Its non-flushing counterpart (niacin as inositol hexanicotinate) reduces the "flushing" side effect caused by niacin, which is similar to hot flashes women have during menopause. Niacin assists in converting food to energy, making hormones, and lowering cholesterol.

A compound made from niacin, Acipimox, has been shown to increase GH in children (treated for dwarfism) and elderly adults. Researchers report, "The data indicates that the decreased GH release associated with aging can be reversed by Acipimox," (*Reduction of free fatty acids by acipimox enhances the growth hormone responses to GH releasing peptide 2 in elderly men*, 2000, Sytze).

High doses of niacin have been shown to be useful in treating high cholesterol. However, side effects can range from flushing to major kidney problems, (*Use of niacin in the prevention and management of hyperlipidemia*, 2001, Robinson). New research shows major problems with niacin supplements and cholesterol-lowering medication. This research is discussed with antioxidants on page 75 of this chapter.

Your Doctor Needs to Know What Supplements You Are Taking

Nutritional supplements always need to be checked for side effects and drug interactions. Niacin (vitamin B-3) reacts with several popular medications, including oral contraceptives, medications to treat cholesterol—Mevacor and Zocor—and oral hypoglycemic agents prescribed for some individuals with Type II diabetes.

A Word About Supplements

Deficiencies in zinc, calcium, potassium, and other minerals significantly deter the release of GH. The need for a good multi-mineral vitamin supplement is clear.

The quality of nutritional supplements is obviously important. And we all know there are those who would make a quick buck selling poor quality supplements, if allowed. For example, some brag about the "USP symbol" placed on their product, as if the product has been lab certified for its high quality. This means that the pill has been tested to dissolve in your stomach. Improvements are being made with supplement ratings. However, it is a good idea to stay with trusted name brands and trusted distributors when shopping for supplements.

Rexall Sundown Inc. was selected Manufacturer of the Year in 2000 by *Nutritional Outlook* magazine, primarily for product quality. Rexall has a Website at www.rexall.com/health called "UniCity Network." Many of their products are sold distributor-direct. And Sundown nutritional products can be purchased at very reasonable retail prices from Wal-Mart.

GNC (owned by the parent company of Rexall Sundown, Royal Numico) has a broad line of products and high standards. GNC prices seem to be reasonable, especially with the "Gold Card" discount.

A trusted independent pharmacist or nutrition store-owner (with an owner-operator you trust), may also be a good source of additional information and savings.

The vitamin-mineral supplement packs from Advocare have produced great results. My wife began using "A Perfect You," multi-mineral-vitamin from Advocare, a few years ago to shed a few pounds and she was pleased with the results. Advocare offers a tasty, low-sugar, energy drink mix called Spark. (*Note:* most energy drinks sold in convenience markets are unfortunately loaded with sugar). On days when I need an extra boost at the gym or the track, Spark does the trick (972-478-4500, or www.advocare.com).

Thermogenic Weight Loss Supplements

Thermogenic supplements claim to increase metabolism and burn calories. And they do, because they increase body heat, which increases metabolism. But there may be side effects, some of which can be serious.

Coffee is a thermogenic agent because it increases body temperature. Products like Diet Fuel, Ripped Fuel, Hydroxycut, and Xenadrine (reported to be the top-selling weight loss supplement in the world) typically contain the herb ma hung, which is ephedrine. These products generally contain some type of herbal caffeine, typically guarana.

While I have never taken Xenadrine, I have two friends that swear by this product, www.xenadrine.com. A close friend lost 35 pounds in three months using Xenadrine—and of course, a new fitness program!

Once, I was cast as a background model for a Xenadrine television commercial—I was the guy in the background admiring the woman that lost weight with the product. During the shooting, I saw the before and after photos of the male and female featured in the commercial. The real life results were almost unbelievable. Based on this experience, I can say that these "before and afters" were not doctored. They both looked great!

I believe there are several good companies selling high quality, beneficial nutritional products. The purpose of this chapter, and this book, is not to recommend nutritional products or their manufacturers. This information is intended to provide general information and is not intended to be product endorsement or medical advice. Decisions concerning nutritional products, health, and any health   related matter should involve consultation with the appropriate medical professional and your physician.

GH "Stacks"- Buyer Beware

GH "stacks" are combinations of amino acids, vitamins, and herbs. The FDA does not regulate stacks as drugs, but as food. And there is a huge difference in regulation of foods versus drugs. The marketing information promoting some of these GH supplement stacks may not be totally up front.

Internet sites sell expensive protein and herb stacks that supposedly promote GH release. If the stacks contain 2 grams of glutamine, then they probably fulfill their claims. However, there may be some real savings opportunity on these supplements. Typically, stacks include amino acids (glutamine, arginine, lysine, and ornithine), vitamins like niacin, and herbs like ginkgo biloba, barrenwort, and others. GH stacks can be expensive. You can easily purchase the key supplements individually for much less, and know that you have research supporting your supplementation plan.

GH Secretagogues

Considerable research is taking place with GH secretagogues. The combination of several amino acids, the first being the development of GHRP-6 (six amino acids) in 1979 by Momany and Bowers at Tulane University, led the way for research into new methods of stimulating GH release. Some manufacturers of GH secretagogues claim that their products are natural. And they are—technically. They are natural in that they are developed with *natural* amino acids. Secretagogues appear to be safer than GH injections. They are also much more complex than single amino acid nutritional supplements.

In *Growth Hormone: Reversing Human Aging Naturally*, James Jamieson recounts his personal involvement in the development of "Symbiotropin," a GH-release agent. This compound utilizes L-dopa, a drug used in the treatment of Parkinson's disease, along with other amino acids and "chaperone molecules."

If you are seriously considering GH-replacement injections for the treatment of GH deficiency, you might want to consider experimenting first with Symbiotropin. Why? GH injections are substitutes. They act *in place of* your body's own GH secretions. Symbiotropin, on the other hand, stimulates your body to manufacture and release GH. This is a huge difference with many ramifications. For example, GH injections may train your pituitary to release less natural growth hormone.

The current medical research concerning GH secretagogues is summarized by Dr. Casabeill and colleagues at the Institute of Endocrinology, Belgrade, Yugoslavia, in *Growth hormone secretagogues: the clinical future* (1999), PubMed abstract:

> *"The combined administration of GH releasing hormone plus GHRP-6, both at saturating doses, is currently the most powerful releaser of GH, devoid of side effects and convenient for the patient; it may also be an alternative to the insulin tolerance test for the diagnosis of GHD in adult patients. Their potential action at cardiovascular level is highly promising. Although the clinical future of GH releasing substances is appealing, probably the most relevant contribution has yet to be discovered."*

The final word on secretagogues is not in yet. And it might be wise to wait for more research before using them except as a first step before GH injections.

Insulin Balance

Insulin and growth hormone are interrelated, as are many hormones. GH does wonderful things for your body, as we have seen. But the balance of insulin in your body can make or break the effects of GH release.

Insulin just may be the most important hormone in controlling energy during fitness training. Insulin has several critical functions in addition to its well-known role of managing excessive sugar consumed in the diet.

Insulin also plays an important role in the control of lipid (fat) metabolism and facilitating the entry of amino acids—the body's building blocks—into muscle. Without an adequate supply of insulin, or with too much insulin (in someone who is insulin resistant), the body's ability to filter sugar from the blood is limited. This condition generally begins in the body as a resistance to insulin, and over time, it may develop into diabetes. Insulin plays a   major role in hypoglycemia, or low blood sugar. Symptoms of this disorder can include breaking out in a cold sweat, dizziness, nausea, light-headedness, and headache.

We need insulin. The key is maintaining the ideal balance of insulin to maximize the benefits of growth hormone. Out of balance insulin levels—high or low—limit GH release.

Individuals with high levels of body fat (usually 30 percent over ideal body weight) often develop a resistance to insulin. "The heavier and more sedentary a patient is, the greater the degree of insulin resistance," (*Syndrome X*, 2001, Reaven). The body reacts by increasing circulating insulin to levels higher than normal. This interferes with GH release and causes a cycle to occur that increases body fat even more.

Researchers at the University of Milano, Milan, Italy, prove that too much insulin stunts GH release.
(Elevated insulin levels contribute to the reduced growth hormone (GH) response to GH-releasing hormone in obese subjects, 1999, Lanzi).

When individuals with insulin resistance eat carbohydrates, normal processes are altered. Carbohydrates do not enter the muscle normally. They go back to the liver and are turned into fat rather than being used for energy. The end result: more body fat and less energy.

"It is the high percentage of body fat relative to lean muscle weight that increases the cells' resistance to insulin," says Nan Allison, licensed nutritionist and author of the highly recommended book *Full & Fulfilled, The Science of Eating to Your Soul's Satisfaction* (800-928-9229 or www.AllisonandBeck.org)

GH release may actually be a function of the balance of insulin levels in your body. You can train for hours, supplement with glutamine, lysine, and arginine, and sleep eight hours. But if you blow it by eating excessive refined sugar (candy and desserts) or too many carbs, causing your insulin level to skyrocket to filter heavy blood sugar, GH release will be restricted.

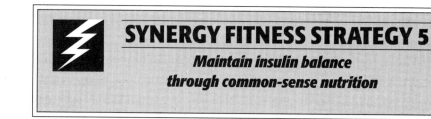

SYNERGY FITNESS STRATEGY 5
Maintain insulin balance through common-sense nutrition

Refined Sugar is the Bad Guy

For a long time, we have known that from the standpoint of extra calories, we pay the price for eating heavy refined sugar such as candy and desserts. But now, here's the double whammy—sugar limits GH secretion.

If you are a high school athlete, you can probably process the extra calories. However, as we age, without GH to keep the fat burning metabolism turned on, weight is gained all too easily.

Not only do high sugar desserts interfere with GH, too much bread, cereal, crackers, and juice relative to the protein in your diet can have the same GH-halting results. People with insulin resistance (often Type II diabetics) are unable to process seemingly "normal" amounts of carbohydrates. Now don't get me wrong, you need carbs in your diet to perform your Strategic Fitness Plan in Chapter 11. Carbs are not evil; in fact, carbs are good. You just need to eat them in moderation.

If you really want to improve health and fitness, enhance appearance, and achieve optimum athletic performance, you must rethink your diet, particularly your consumption of refined sugar.

The Atkins Diet has been very successful for many. In an interview discussing the basic principles of his diet, Dr. Atkins said, "Fat doesn't make you fat, sugar does." When you understand how GH and insulin function, this makes sense.

Carbs and calories must be severely restricted if you are not active in fitness training. Otherwise, body weight will continue to increase and so will insulin resistance. However, high intensity fitness training will help to compensate for eating some on-the-go meals.

Insulin resistance can be improved by weight loss, balanced diet, and moderate-intensity exercise. (Insulin action after resistive training in insulin resistant older men and women, 2001, Ryan).

Exercise Improves Insulin Resistance

Resistance to insulin occurs mostly in overweight individuals. This is a serious medical condition and is usually the first step toward diabetes, hypertension, high cholesterol, and cardiovascular disease.

Insulin resistance syndrome occurs long before these diseases appear. And it occurs mostly in adults with abdominal obesity, general obesity, and family history. It also occurs in older adults who have lost muscular strength, (*Insulin resistance syndrome*, 2001, Rao). This is why adults over ninety have seen great results in clinical trials with weight training.

Researchers at Brigham and Women's Hospital in Boston measured the impact of being overweight (not obese, just overweight) on developing serious diseases. The researchers conclude that the risk for chronic diseases (heart disease, colon cancer, diabetes) is approximately twenty times higher for overweight people. And the risks for serious diseases increases relative to the degree individuals are overweight, (*Impact of overweight on the risk of developing common chronic diseases during a 10-year period*, 2001, Field).

Degrees of Health and Fitness

The following discussion concerning diabetes and hypoglycemia is directly related to sugar in the diet. The treatment for both of these conditions is the same—avoid sugar, lose "fat" weight (lose fat and keep muscle), and exercise regularly.

Since many adults have not been diagnosed with either condition (yet), they feel they are operating within a healthy range. However, the absence of illness does not necessarily mean an individual is healthy.

Many middle-aged Americans may be closer than they think to being diagnosed with diabetes. There are 8 million undiagnosed cases today, and 650,000 Americans will learn they have diabetes this year.

Between the extremes of diabetes and hypoglycemia, there are several levels of wellness. And the potential to reach optimum wellness. Do not be satisfied with resting at borderline wellness when you can change course. Set your goal for optimum fitness, not just the absence of disease.

> *Vitamin E is associated with improved insulin action.* (Vitamin E, vitamin C, and exercise, 2000, Evans).

Diabetes–A Disease of Middle Age

Diabetes is a disease caused by the inability of the pancreas to produce high enough levels of insulin, a hormone that helps the body absorb glucose (sugar) into the cells where it can be used as an energy source. Without the appropriate amount of insulin, the body's supply of sugar continues to build in the blood and urine. And the kidneys become unable to filter the excessive sugar. The results: weakness, fatigue, blurred vision, irritability, and excessive thirst, hunger and urination.

Diabetes is the seventh leading cause of death in the United States, and only half of the 16 million Americans with diabetes have been diagnosed. Untreated, diabetes can result in blindness; amputation of the toe, foot, or leg; kidney dialysis; and eventually, death.

The great news is that most diabetics can be successfully treated with weight loss, a sugar-free diet, and serious fitness training. The Strategic Fitness Plan, Level One, prescribed in Chapter 11 is suitable as a starter program (with physician approval) for diabetic patients.

The most severe cases of diabetes (Type I) representing 5 to 10 percent of diagnosed cases, are treated with insulin injections coupled with diet, exercise, and weight loss. (CDC).

Clinical Alert: Diet and Exercise Dramatically Delay Type II Diabetes

This announcement was made in August 2001 by Health and Human Services Secretary Tommy Thompson at the National Institutes of Health. The full report can be viewed at www.nlm.nih.gov/databases/alerts/diabetes01.html.

Hypoglycemia

The symptoms of hypoglycemia are weakness, shakiness, anxiety, faintness, and personality and mood change. Because of the nature of these symptoms, hypoglycemia is often misdiagnosed as a mood/mental problem rather than a physiological problem—low blood sugar. Hypoglycemia can be an overdose reaction to insulin injections.

A milder form of this disease, "reactive" hypoglycemia, can be spontaneously induced by stress mixed with a high dose of sugar. For example—someone on a fad starvation diet encounters a stressful situation and decides to blow the diet with a candy bar. Without protein or fat in the system, the pancreas shoots insulin into the bloodstream to counteract the sugar. The person gets giddy for a few moments and then begins to feel weak and even tremble. A diet lower in carbohydrates and higher in protein typically controls the reactive form of hypoglycemia.

Resources: The American Diabetes Association, www.diabetes.org

National Institute of Diabetes & Digestive & Kidney diseases, www.niddk.nih.gov

Achieving Insulin Balance for the Highest Degree of Health and Fitness

Insulin balance in your body is very important. Not only to protect against the diseases caused by extreme insulin imbalances (diabetes and hypoglycemia) but also to achieve the highest degree of health and fitness possible.

Growth hormone is rendered void by too much or too little insulin. With too little insulin, GH cannot facilitate its growth functions of building muscle and body support structure. With too much insulin, GH release shuts down.

To achieve the highest level of fitness, your goal should be to maintain the ideal balance of insulin, blood sugar, and body fat. How? Use the same strategy that applies to increasing growth hormone—a balanced diet (with limited sugar) in moderation, appropriate sleep, GH-release-enhancing nutritional supplements, and a strategic fitness plan that includes high-intensity anaerobic training.

> *Growth hormone is reduced when insulin levels are elevated.* (Elevated *insulin levels contribute to the reduced growth hormone response to GH-releasing hormone in obese subjects,* 1999, Lanzi).

High-Intensity Training Creates Synergy by Producing Antioxidant Benefits

High-intensity fitness training increases growth hormone naturally. And this level of exercise intensity yields other key health benefits, including antioxidant benefits. Antioxidants play a huge role in health and wellness by scavenging the blood for free radical cells, which have been linked to cancer. Some free radical cells are needed to fight disease and heal injury. However, when the body is exposed to environmental pollutants, free radicals are produced in excess.

High-intensity exercise that produces lactate may need to be considered "antioxidant agents" because of its ability to scavenge for oxygen (O2) free radicals. (Free radical scavenging and antioxidant effects of lactate ion: an in vitro study, 2000, Groussard). Achieving the "lactic acid threshold" during exercise has numerous benefits in addition to the impact on GH release.

Excessive free radicals cause damage and leave the body more susceptible to carcinogens. Free radicals play a role in heart disease and hardening of the arteries when they oxidize combined with the low-density (bad) cholesterol.

The damage is actually done by the oxidation of free radicals. Oxidation in the blood operates in the same way that metal oxidizes (when left outside in the weather). When metal tarnishes, it is being oxidized. That's what excessive free radical reactions do in your bloodstream.

The traditional approach to combat free radicals has been to increase the amount of food rich in vitamins C, E, beta-carotene (orange fruit and vegetables—carrots, sweet potatoes), and selenium, and take antioxidant supplements.

Researchers in Finland report that aerobic and anaerobic exercise both produce small amounts of free radicals. (Remember that it is the "excessive" free radicals that do the damage.) The free radicals produced during exercise "insults heart muscle." But this is actually positive. The "insult" causes the heart to develop an "adaptive response" that builds antioxidant defenses into heart muscle, (*Physical exercise and antioxidant defenses in the heart*, 1999, Atalay).

Since high-intensity anaerobic exercise actually causes production of some free radicals to heal muscle tissue, I take a strong, mega-dose, vitamin-mineral supplement (mega-dose, not overdose) containing C, E, beta-carotene, and selenium in the mornings and again after a workout, or during the evening.

Like everything in health, fitness, diet, and nutrition, the keys to success are balance and moderation. New research from the department of Endocrinology at the University of Washington shows that antioxidant supplements actually block the clinical ability of niacin and a drug class called "statins" (simvastatin-niacin) to treat cholesterol problems, (Cheung, 2001).

Don't rely on medications alone to keep you healthy. The research findings concerning statins were unexpected. Statins treat cholesterol problems for 12 million people. Many thought that they could continue to have poor eating habits, remain overweight, and operate without a fitness program by simply taking a pill (one of the statin drugs) to cover the damage caused by poor cholesterol numbers.

Now we see the Public Citizen's Health Research Group petitioning the Food and Drug Administration to add warnings for statins (Mevacor, Zocor, Lescol, and Lipitor) because of the risk of rhabdomyolysis (a rare condition that breaks down muscle tissue). Bayer even pulled its statin (Baycol), after 31 deaths from rhabdomyolysis, *(FDA urged to beef up statin warning,* 2001).

On top of this bad news for individuals with cholesterol problems, *USA Today* reports that new government guidelines concerning cholesterol measurements mean that one in five adults should be taking medication for high cholesterol.

This report means that there are 23 million more people that should be taking medications like statins for cholesterol problems. But new research shows that statins have serious side effects. And another study shows that beneficial antioxidant supplements may block the effectiveness of the statins class of medication.

Many Americans who were thought to have acceptable levels of LDL, the artery-clogging "bad" cholesterol, are now considered to have excessive levels. (More people need cholesterol drugs, USA Today, May, 16, 2001).

Calculate the impact of your cholesterol values on your risk of a heart attack during the next 10 years at: http:// hin.nhlbi.nih.gov/ atpiii/calculator.asp

This research leads to two conclusions: (1) Don't rely solely on medications to keep you healthy; (2) A comprehensive fitness plan that includes adequate sleep, a balanced diet in moderation, appropriate nutritional supplements, and a strategic fitness plan designed to achieve lasting results will provide many health and wellness benefits.

Conclusion

Staying youthful in appearance and rediscovering the energy of your youth lies within the strategy for increasing the number and intensity of growth hormone pulse releases in your body. The key to achieving superior athletic performance is increasing GH release during off-season training. And the key to reversing the somatopause phase of middle age is increasing the natural release of GH in your body. Based on the information in this chapter, I hope you will commit to the following action plan provided on the next page.

New levels of health, fitness, and appearance are realistic goals. Increasing synergistic growth hormone naturally provides many positive benefits—improved health and fitness, increased energy, enhanced productivity, improved appearance, better self-esteem, and better sleep. Make the commitment today to implement a strategic fitness plan for the initial eight weeks.

IMMEDIATE STRATEGIES TO INCREASE GROWTH HORMONE NATURALLY

1. I will make the commitment to follow a Strategic Fitness Plan in Chapter 11.   YES_____ NO_____

2. I will limit refined sugar in my diet—especially two to three hours after training.   YES_____ NO_____

3. I will reorganize my sleeping conditions to increase deep slow wave sleep.   YES_____ NO_____

4. I will consider GH release enhancing supplements—protein supplements and L-glutamine.   YES_____ NO_____

5. I will work on coping with stress.   YES_____ NO_____

6. I will say no to GH replacement injections until the above strategies are no longer effective (should be around age 90).   YES_____ NO_____

7. I will ask my physician for advice about any part of this book, should I have questions.   YES_____ NO_____

4

The Target Zone Training Method

Understanding how to increase growth hormone (GH) in your body through exercise; and getting the absolute most benefit from your fitness training time, requires a basic understanding of the how your body creates energy, and how your muscles operate.

Basically, you have three types of muscle fiber, and three different systems in your body that generate energy. The three types of muscle fiber and the three energy systems are made to work together for your benefit...that is, if you'll work them through the right kind of exercise.

Your body has one type of slow-twitch muscle fiber, and two types of fast-twitch muscle fiber–type IIa, and the super fast IIx. Type IIa muscle moves five times faster than the slow-twitch muscle, and the super fast IIx moves 10 times faster.

It's important to know about these two systems and why you need to regularly exercise all three types of muscle fibers and develop the three energy systems in your body.

Most people quit exercising their fast-twitch muscles when they stop competitive sports. This is unfortunate because it's this type of exercise that causes your body to significantly increase it's own production of GH...naturally.

Heads Up—About This Chapter

The discussions in this chapter concerning the Target Zone Training Method are, quite frankly, complex. But I will attempt to simplify these concepts. Understanding how the body's energy systems relate to the body's muscle fiber composition may be hard work on your part, perhaps requiring backing up and rereading a section. The reward for your effort in taking some extra time to understand these concepts will result in the knowledge you need to improve athletic performance, delay the middle age somatopause, and reverse the effects of aging by as much as 20 years. It's worth the effort!

How Your Body Generates Energy

The body's energy systems relate to how the body generates its two main sources of energy—energy from the diet, and energy from the air we breathe.

The three energy systems in the body operate somewhat like a car with three gears. The first gear is called "ATP-PC," second gear is "anaerobic lactate," and third gear is called "aerobic."

The body shifts to one of these three energy systems depending on the level of work or exercise intensity.

Just like gas for your car, your body is fueled by energy produced by (1) the oxygen you breathe, and (2) your diet—carbohydrates (sugar glucose) and fat (cholesterol and triglycerides). Even though protein is the building block of muscle, protein is not burned for energy except in cases of starvation or extreme exhaustion, such as "hitting the wall" at the 20 mile point in a marathon.

Fuel sources from the diet are digested and transported to the blood system for potential energy use. When your body needs energy, it takes glucose from the diet and combines it with oxygen in the blood. This combination becomes "glycogen" (glucose + oxygen). It is stored in your muscles so it will be immediately available to burn for quick-bursts of energy. And just like driving in first gear, this process uses lots of fuel...fast.

During exercise, your stored glycogen and sugar glucose in the blood convert to ATP (adenosine triphosphate), and this gives your muscles the energy to move.

An easy way to understand this process is to think of carbohydrates and fats in your diet as firewood and ATP as the fire. ATP burns all its energy within 1 or 2 seconds and is refueled by the body in three different ways, depending on the intensity of the exercise.

It's important to note that ATP can only burn as energy when it has fuel to burn. And oxygen is a key source of fuel. When there is plenty of oxygen available, aerobic processes continually supply fuel. However, when the exercise is high-intensity like sprinting, and there is not enough oxygen available for fuel, stored fuel sources can only make enough ATP to last for 6 to 8 seconds. This is an anaerobic (without oxygen) condition. And this is also a fundamental GH release benchmark that you need to achieve during fitness training.

Researchers report "metabolic fuel" during fitness training (the way the body burns energy during exercise) and "tissue repair after exercise" play important roles in growth hormone release. (Exercise and growth hormone: does one affect the other?" 1997, Roemmich).

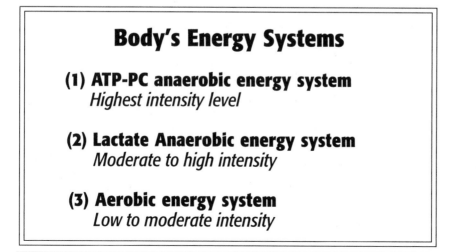

Body's Energy Systems

(1) ATP-PC anaerobic energy system
Highest intensity level

(2) Lactate Anaerobic energy system
Moderate to high intensity

(3) Aerobic energy system
Low to moderate intensity

Energy for Exercise–Phase 1: ATP-PC

Exercise achieving the highest level of intensity uses the *ATP-PC anaerobic* energy system. ATP-PC is characterized by a short-burst type of effort. This type of exercise is so fast and demanding that it causes an insufficient supply of oxygen in the blood.

Even though there is insufficient oxygen to supply energy, the body is able to meet energy demands by producing a new compound (ATP-PC) as fuel to burn. But the body can only do this for up to 6 to 8 seconds, the approximate time it takes to sprint 50 to 70-yards.

During the first 8 seconds of high intensity anaerobic exercise, ATP begins burning energy so quickly it cannot get enough oxygen. ATP then combines with *phosphocreatine (PC),* which is stored in muscle cells for quick, maximal type of energy demands. The purpose of ATP-PC is to fuel the body's quick-burst, high-intensity energy demands without oxygen. And while anaerobic exercise may feel unnatural, your body was made to handle this level of intensity.

At the cellular level, ATP-PC temporarily robs oxygen from the body, and the "oxygen debt" must be paid back immediately. Cells must breathe oxygen (cellular respiration) or die. Anyone who has sprinted or walked quickly up several flights of stairs, has felt oxygen debt.

At the end of an 8 to 12 second 60-meter sprint, it takes huge intakes of air to pay back oxygen debt. Cells are seeking oxygen for all the muscles that worked during the sprint. While this is slightly painful, this type of quick-burst, out-of-breath, type of exercise can do wonderful things for your body.

The anaerobic 60-meter (70-yards) sprint that causes oxygen debt and the "burning"sensation from lactic acid build-up, also stimulates the pituitary to release anti-aging, anti–middle aging, performance-improving growth hormone. Oxygen debt payback is unpleasant, but it is an important barometer for GH-releasing exercise. Medical research clearly demonstrates that ATP-PC anaerobic exercise produces the largest release of GH in direct relation to the intensity of exercise, (Pritzlaff, 2000).

Energy for Exercise–Phase 2: Anaerobic Lactate

Exercise at the 70 percent intensity range triggers a different cellular metabolism than the ATP-PC, first gear. Second gear, anaerobic lactate, begins when the ATP-PC have been burned, and the body continues to burn glucose and some limited oxygen. This process can supply energy needs at the exercise intensity rate of 70 to 90 percent for 30 to 60 seconds.

The by-products of the ATP-PC and anaerobic lactate energy systems are lactic acid and hydrogen ions in the muscles, which cause muscles to become acidic and painful. The lactic acid actually begins aggravating the nerve endings in the muscles–and causes sensations of pain.

Anaerobic exercise can be slightly painful, and it can be dangerous. Warning: Anaerobic exercise is typically necessary to increase GH from exercise, but it can also be dangerous to someone with heart problems. If you have any question about your health, or your ability to perform this type of exercise, see your physician BEFORE attempting anaerobic fitness training.

Researchers show a direct correlation of GH release with a wide variety of anaerobic and high-intensity aerobic exercise–from weightlifting to cycling, with fit and unfit men. There are "linear correlations" between GH release and "oxygen demand and availability." In short, you need to reach the out-of-breath stage to release GH. (Regulation of growth hormone during exercise by oxygen demand and availability, 1987, Vanhelder).

Running 150-meters to 400-meters (440-yards or one lap around the track) above 80 percent intensity will not only cause oxygen debt, but also produce slight pain in the muscles. The body's reaction to the stress of anaerobic exercise may trigger adrenal involvement, which is also responsible for GH release through secretion of adrenaline.

This level of intensity can be accomplished by exercise in the first two gears—ATP-PC, or the anaerobic lactate gear, but typically not in the aerobic gear.

The greater the intensity of exercise, the greater the release of GH. The 20-minute Sprint 8 Workout described in Chapter 8 will provide an efficient way of achieving this goal within a limited time frame. The Sprint 8 Workout intensity level is based on age and current fitness level, so do not let the discussion of sprinting deter your enthusiasm for the benefits of anaerobic exercise.

You could sprint 200 to 400-meters at 80 percent intensity and reach the lactate gear (depending on your age and conditioning) to accomplish GH release benchmarks. In fact, to add additional intensity to GH release exercise programs for Fitness Level Five—college and professional athletes—the top level of intensity offers the option of adding longer sprints. However, the Sprint 8 Workout (with varying levels of intensity) is the basic routine for all Fitness Levels—and it can be completed in only 20 minutes.

Energy to Exercise–Phase 3: Aerobic

When the body supplies energy aerobically—with a steady supply of oxygen in the blood fueling ATP (due to low-intensity exercise)—the *aerobic* system, or third gear, is engaged. Carbs and fats supplying fuel for this energy system will eventually give out before the oxygen fuel source is depleted. Aerobic low-intensity walking, jogging, and swimming are examples of aerobic exercise.

Researchers show that lactic acid levels and corresponding GH levels are "significant" in anaerobic exercise versus aerobic exercise, (*Effects of anaerobic and aerobic exercise of equal duration and work expenditure on plasma growth hormone levels*, Vanhelder, 1984). The exception is aerobic exercise that borderlines anaerobic and stays above the lactate threshold for 30 minutes. This level of intensity also stimulates GH release, (Wideman, 1999). An example would be a demanding 30-minute run at a 75 percent intensity level.

Aerobic exercise, often called "cardio," is the mainstay of many fitness programs. Aerobic exercise is great for burning calories, building the endurance base necessary for most sports, and maintaining wellness. The principle behind aerobic exercise is reaching the "target heart rate" (calculated by an age-specific formula) and maintaining that heart rate for 20 to 30 minutes.

The Sprint 8 Workout achieves GH release and aerobic target rate for the duration of the 20 minute program. How? With each of the eight sprint repetitions, heart rate is sent racing far above the aerobic target rate. During the 1.5 to 2-minute (walk-back to the start) recovery between each sprint, the heart rate remains at, or above, the aerobic target rate. In other words, you will train all three energy systems, including the aerobic energy system with the Sprint 8 Workout.

> *Researchers demonstrate that aerobic exercise below the lactate threshold does not increase GH, whereas, "GH is significantly elevated after only 10 minutes of high-intensity exercise."* (Effect of low and high intensity exercise on circulating growth hormone in men, 1992, Felsing).

SYNERGY FITNESS STRATEGY 6
Use GH-releasing exercise targeting the body's three energy systems

Training All Three Muscle Fiber Types

It is impossible to train all three muscle fiber types by accident. The *Target Zone Method* is a fitness strategy that targets the body's three energy systems during training and this method also targets the specific muscle fiber types—fast-twitch types IIa and the super fast IIx, and slow-twitch muscles.

The Target Zone Method of training has far-reaching benefits. The reason? Fast-twitch muscle development is not only vitally important to competitive athletes, researchers now show that this form of exercise may delay, and even reverse, the effects of aging, and middle aging.

Developing Slow-Twitch Muscle Fiber

Type I muscle fibers are called "slow-twitch" because they contract slower than IIa and IIx muscles. Type I fibers operate in the third aerobic gear.

> ## Slow-twitch muscles are in large supply in the body, and are supplied with oxygen by many capillaries.

This muscle itself is red (perhaps from being rich with blood) and is the main muscle group used in aerobic endurance training. Aerobic exercise like jogging, and walking, and the traditional methods of weightlifting, normally develops slow-twitch type I muscle.

Developing Fast-Twitch IIa Muscle Fiber

Type IIa fibers are called "fast oxidative" because these red muscles have a great supply of capillaries to supply them with blood. Type IIa is resistant to fatigue like slow-twitch muscle fiber. However, these muscle fibers move approximately 5 times faster than slow-twitch muscles. Type IIa fiber is used during moderate to high-intensity exercise and matches with the exercise that targets the second gear–anaerobic lactate energy system.

Fitness programs targeting IIa muscle fiber would include interval training of 30 to 60 seconds. Some plyometrics, Olympic lifting, and weight-plyos (Chapter 9) target the IIa muscle fiber, and may work the super fast IIx fast-twitch muscle.

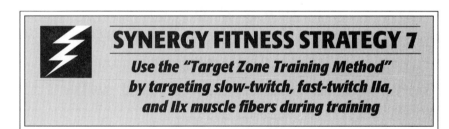

SYNERGY FITNESS STRATEGY 7

Use the "Target Zone Training Method" by targeting slow-twitch, fast-twitch IIa, and IIx muscle fibers during training

Developing Fast-Twitch IIx Muscle Fiber

Fast-twitch IIx (sometimes called IIb) is officially called "fast glycolytic" because it burns energy from stored glycogen for quick-burst. Type IIx muscle fiber aligns with the **first gear, ATP-PC energy system.**

Type IIx has relatively few capillaries to supply the muscle with blood (perhaps this is why the muscle is white). This super fast muscle fiber moves 10 times faster than slow-twitch and 5 times faster than fast-twitch IIa muscle fiber. Exercising type IIx muscle fiber is critical in increasing GH from exercise.

> ## Type IIx muscle specializes in scoring touchdowns, winning gold metals in the Olympics, delaying the middle age somatopause, and reversing the effects of aging by 20 years.

The Ten Synergy Fitness Strategies and the Strategic Fitness Plans, in this book, contain specific strategies and workouts aimed a Target Zones in your body—your body's three energy systems and three muscle fiber types.

With weight training for example, the Target Zones are the major body parts and the three types of fiber within each group.

"Zoning In" and Hitting the Target

The following table outlines the alignment of muscle fiber types, the body's energy systems, and intensity levels. This table shows the type of fitness training that is required to zone-in on the target and work muscle fiber types while simultaneously hitting your body's three energy systems.

Targeting Muscle Types During Fitness Training

TARGET: MUSCLE TYPES	IIX	IIA	I
Target: ENERGY SYSTEMS	ATP-PC	anaerobic lactate	aerobic
speed	fast	medium	slow
muscle color	white	red	red
capillaries	few	many	many
oxygen capacity	low	medium	high
Zoning in: type of training	anaerobic: Sprint 8 (8 reps of 70 yards)	anaerobic: plyo-weights, plyometrics 150m sprints	aerobic: 20-30 minutes -Cardio
Zoning in: intensity of training	90% - 95%	75% - 90%	50% - 75%

Your Body's Composition of Muscle Fiber Types—Half Slow, Half Fast

The average person has approximately 50 percent fast-twitch (IIa and IIx) and 50 percent slow twitch (type I) fiber. However, there can be swings in fiber composition, (*Muscle, Genes, and Athletic Performance*, September 2000, Scientific American, Jesper).

Sprinters have more of all three fiber types than average, and a higher percentage of fast IIx. Endurance trained individuals have more slow type I.

The following chart demonstrates that while there are differences in fiber composition, there is approximately a 50/50 split (with deviations of 10 percent or so) between fast-twitch and slow-twitch fibers.

Muscle Fiber Composition

	Average	Sprint trained	Aerobic trained
Slow type I	40%	40%	55%
Fast type IIa	50%	20%	40%
Fast type IIx	10%	40%	5%

Although there are differences in muscle fiber composition, it is easy to conclude that regardless of one's sport or training emphasis—anaerobic, aerobic, or in between—a comprehensive training approach targeting the three muscle fiber types and three energy systems would be beneficial. **It might also be reasonable to conclude that 50 percent of your training time should be on slow-twitch exercise (cardio, weights), 30 percent on IIa exercises (weight-plyos, intervals), and 20 percent on IIx exercises (sprints).**

Muscle Fiber Activation Process

The intensity of exercise determines the activation level of different fiber types. In a low-intensity demand on the body, the brain tells only the slow type I muscle fiber to respond to meet the demand. In a moderate-intensity demand, type IIa fast-twitch fiber responds along with the slow fiber. And during high-intensity demand, type IIx muscle fiber responds with the other fibers.

Researchers show that GH release is tied to high-intensity exercise (Chapters 1–3). And a comprehensive fitness improvement strategy should include anaerobic (GH-releasing) exercise as well as resistance training, aerobic "cardio" work to build endurance, and flexibility training. The major components of a total fitness approach are discussed in the following chapter.

Conclusion

CONGRATULATIONS! You have successfully completed the *Ready* phase of *Ready, Set, GO!* The next section will get you *Set* and prepared for the action phase that begins in the *GO* section.

The *Set* section contains a chapter for each of the major components of Synergy Fitness and an introductory chapter (coming up next) describing how to build your Strategic Fitness Plan.

Without a comprehensive fitness plan that targets the three muscle fiber types, an individual could actually be exercising only half of his or her muscles. "There was a significant increase in the proportion of type II fibers," researchers report. "Our results are encouraging in that they suggest an effect of growth hormone on a specific aging-correlated deficit." (Growth hormone administration and exercise effects on muscle fiber type and diameter in moderately frail older people, 2001, Hennessey).

Building Your Strategic Fitness Plan

THIS CHAPTER BEGINS THE SET PHASE of "Ready, Set, GO!" It will show you how to build your Strategic Fitness Plan.

Your Strategic Fitness Plan has five major parts —flexibility, endurance, strength, power, and anaerobic training. Regardless of your age and current physical condition, your fitness plan should have planned workouts addressing every major area of fitness.

All of these areas do not need to be exercise daily. In fact, major muscle groups typically need 48 hours to recover. And most injuries are simply "overuse injuries" that can take months to heal–so the frequency of your training needs to be carefully programmed into your fitness plan. For these reasons, a weekly perspective of fitness training is ideal.

A good rule of thumb: most fitness components need training two times a week, while some areas—endurance, flexibility, and anaerobic training—need more frequent work. The following chart outlines ideal training frequency by fitness component.

MAJOR COMPONENTS OF A STRATEGIC FITNESS PLAN

Fitness Component:	Type of training	Time requirement	Training frequency	Fiber type	Energy system
Flexibility *Chapter 6*	Stretching	10 minutes	3-4 x week	All fibers	Aerobic
Endurance *Chapter 7*	Cardio	Target heart rate for 20 minutes	2-3 x week *-may be multi-tasked with anaerobic training*	Slow type I	Aerobic
Anaerobic *Chapter 8*	Sprint 8 -run, swim, cycle, skate	20 minutes	2-3 x week	IIx	ATP-PC
Power *Chapter 9*	Plyometrics Plyo-weights	10-20 minutes First 30 percent of reps	1 x week Every weight workout	IIa IIa & IIx	Lactate ATP-PC
Strength *Chapter 10*	Weight training *-Classical gym type strength training*	30-60 minutes	3-4 x week	Slow type I	Aerobic

To get the full effect of Synergy Fitness, the benchmarks for growth hormone release—muscle burn (lactic acid), oxygen debt, rising body temperature, and adrenal response (Chapter 1) need to occur on as many training days as possible. All components of Synergy Fitness are not designed to achieve GH release. However, all fitness components are necessary.

Flexibility and endurance training, for example, will typically not reach the GH release threshold. However, without adequate flexibility and an energizing endurance base developed by aerobic training, it would be difficult to perform the other fitness programs that actually increase GH.

Specific workouts are illustrated in the following five chapters—one chapter for each major component of Synergy Fitness. For the anaerobic component, the "Sprint 8 Workout" is described, and the "10-Minute Stretching Routine" is recommended for the flexibility component. These workouts will be scheduled into weekly training plans programmed for the five different levels of fitness discussed in this chapter.

To illustrate how this works, the Level Two Strategic Fitness Plan for Week 1 will be used as the example. For every Fitness Level (One through Five) there is a highlighted outline called the **Exercise Prescription**. This overview guide shows the training plan for a full week of comprehensive training.

The Strategic Fitness Plans for the first four weeks of training follow the Exercise Prescription. These plans have the specific information of what needs to be done during every workout.

"100 percent of the age-related decline in aerobic power among middle aged men occurring over 30 years was reversed by six months of endurance training." A 30-year follow-up of the Dallas bedrest and training study: II. Effect of age on cardiovascular adaptation to exercise training, 2001, McGuire).

STRATEGIC FITNESS PLAN
Exercise Prescription - Level Two

MONDAY	TUESDAY	WEDNESDAY	THURSDAY	FRIDAY	SATURDAY	SUNDAY
10-Minute Stretching Routine *Chapter 6*	**Weights** 1 hour *Chapter 10*		**10-Minute Stretching Routine**	**10-Minute Stretching Routine**	**Weights** 1 hour	**Rest**
Sprint 8 20 minutes *Chapter 8*	**Cardio-20** 20 minutes *Chapter 7*	*Make up day*	**Weights** 1 hour	**Sprint 8**		
				Plyometrics *Chapter 9*		**TOTAL WEEK TIME:** 4 hours 45 mins
30 minutes	1 hour 20 minutes		1 hour 10 minutes	45 minutes	1 hour	

Exercising at home is just as effective as at a gym. (Effects of intermittent exercise and the use of home exercise equipment adherence, weight loss, and fitness in overweight women: A random trial, 1999, Jakicic).

Workouts differ day by day in the training schedule to allow muscle groups adequate rest. Wednesday is the planned make up day for Level Two. Should work interfere with your fitness plan for the week, you can use this day for catch-up.

Notice the time allocation for the Level Two fitness plan—less than five hours weekly (and less than three and a half hours for Level One). In the time it takes to play one round of golf or watch a couple of movies, you can complete a week of comprehensive fitness training that will dramatically improve your health, fitness, and appearance.

Get your week started right. Make Monday a good workout day. Mondays are the heaviest days in most fitness centers (no research on this, just a personal observation over 30 years). And Mondays are hectic, but I have found that a good workout on Monday sets the pace for the entire week. Give Monday's workout your best effort, and the remainder of the week will fall in place!

In the time it takes to watch a couple of movies, you can complete a week of comprehensive fitness training that will dramatically improve your health, fitness and appearance.

Tracking Success with Your Strategic Fitness Training Log

The Strategic Fitness Plan is also a Training Log is for tracking your success. By charting and writing fitness progress in your Training Log every workout, you can track the success you are experiencing and set goals for the following workout. Motivation to continue high-intensity exercise is related to positive outcomes, and you will be seeing positive results quickly with this fitness plan.

Your Training Log contains a workbook section to record the amount of resistance (weight) used during weightlifting. The key to success with fitness training is to plan you work, and work the plan, and record your results. Charting results with fitness training yields greater success.

The Strategic Fitness Plans are designed to attack one day and one week at a time. At the beginning of the week, plan your training schedule for the entire week. And before every workout, spend a couple of minutes reviewing your previous performance and mentally preparing for the workout.

A sample of a Strategic Fitness Plan and Training Log— Level Two, Week 1 follows. This is what a completed Training Log should look like at the end of the first week of training.

STRATEGIC FITNESS PLAN

Training Log   Level Two   Week 1   Date_____

Workout:	Training Plan:	M	T	W	Th	F	Sat	S
10-Minute Stretching	**3 x week (M, Th, F)** *Chapter 6*	X			X	X		
Cardio *Chapter 7*	**30 minutes 1 x week** *Tuesday or Thursday*		30 mins					
Sprint 8 *Chapter 8*	**20 minutes 2 x week** *30-50% speed/intensity during first 4 weeks. 8 reps 70-yards, walk back.*	6 70s				8 70s		
Plyometrics *Chapter 9*	**15 minutes 1 x week** *1 set plyo-drills at half-speed*					X		

Weight Training:	Exercise: *Chapter 10*	Record Sets & Reps Performance *sets/reps*			Record amount of weight used during sets in shaded areas. **NOTE: Perform weight-plyo techniques (Chapter 9) on first 3 to 5 reps per set.**				
Chest	Bench press 2/12	2/12	2/12	2/10	100		105	105	
	Incline press 1/12	1/12	1/12	1/10	70		75	80	
	Chest stretch 30 sec	X	X	X					
Back	Pull downs 2/12	2/12	2/15	2/10	90		90	95	
	Up back stretch 30 sec	X	X	X					
Shoulders	Shoulder press 2/10	2/10	2/12	2/15	80		80	80	
	Front laterals 1/10	1/10	1/10	1/14	12		15	15	
	Shrugs 1/20	1/10	1/20	1/20	20		20	25	
	Shoulder stretch 30 sec	X	X	X					
	Rotator cuff 1/15	1/10	1/12	1/15	15		15	15	
Biceps	Curls 2/10	2/12	2/15	2/10	15		15	15	
	Incline DB curl 1/10	1/10	1/12	1/12	15		15	15	
Triceps	Press downs 3/20	3/15	3/18	3/20	60		70	70	
Quads	Leg press 2/20	2/20	2/23	2/20	70		80	80	
	Leg ext 1/20	1/20	1/20	1/16	60		60	70	
Hamstrings	Leg curls 1/15	1/14	1/15	1/18	40		40	40	
Calves	3-way calf raises 1/21	1/21	1/21	1/21	100		100	100	
Abs	Leg raises 1/20	20	22	23					
	Crunches 1/25	25	25	25					
Obliques	Twists 1/20	20	20	20					

Age, Current Fitness Level, and Training Experience Determine Your Starting Level

There are five levels built into the Strategic Fitness Plans in Chapter 11. You need to place yourself in one of the five categories. When in doubt, place yourself in the lower level initially—you can always move up to the next level.

- **Level One**—newcomers, those not exercising regularly, adults over age 60, and children 14 and under.

- **Level Two**—adults who have been exercising, but not with comprehensive training or with high-intensity workouts; and adults age 40 to 70. There is some overlapping with ages due to variables in fitness levels.

- **Level Three**—physically fit individuals, at any age, who are active in a single aspect of fitness, such as distance running, weight training, or bodybuilding. Even for the experienced and physically fit, individuals entering at this Level need to keep in mind that new dimensions of training should be added incrementally.

- **Level Four**—advanced physically fit individuals ages 18 to 40 experienced in high-intensity training.

- **Level Five**—college and professional athletes.

> *Researchers report "vigorous activities" and "total physical activity" show the strongest reduction in coronary heart disease. Moderate and light activities are "nonsignificant" in reducing the risk of heart disease. (Physical activity and coronary heart disease in men: The Harvard Alumni Health Study, 2000, Sesso).*

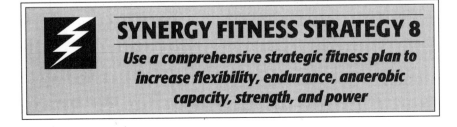

SYNERGY FITNESS STRATEGY 8
Use a comprehensive strategic fitness plan to increase flexibility, endurance, anaerobic capacity, strength, and power

Researchers found that men at age 65 can achieve a hormonal response during training equal to younger men—if the exercise is similar in intensity.
(Hormonal responses to maximal and submaximal exercise in trained and untrained men of various ages, 1996, Silverman).

AGE AND CURRENT FITNESS LEVEL

Fitness program	Level One	Level Two	Level Three	Level Four	Level Five
Current fitness level	Inactive, just starting	Healthy, moderate fitness level	Fit	Very fit	Superb fitness level
Training experience	New comer	Exercising some, but little high intensity	Exercising regularly	Experienced	College or Pro athlete
Age	Over 60 Under 14	30-70	30-50	18-40	18-30

What Time of Day to Train?

What's the best time for fitness training? This is a frequent question. Research shows that any time of day is okay as long as you get the job done . . . with intensity!

A recent study shows that time of day is not a factor in increasing GH release during fitness training, *(Cortisol and growth hormone response to exercise at different times of day,* 2001, Kanaley). Careful not to train too late at night because this can impact sleep.

Strategic Fitness Training and Aging

At any age, a comprehensive approach to improving fitness is clearly the correct approach. Otherwise, as much as 50 percent of muscle fiber in the body's muscle composition could remain untouched during training (Chapter 4).

As we age, activity that once developed (and maintained) fast-twitch muscle fiber lessens (or disappears), and so do these muscle fibers. Although slow-twitch muscle fiber may be developed even in older ages, if fast-twitch fiber is not equally developed during aging, fitness progress will be limited. Not using fast-twitch muscles during aging essentially means that these fibers (as much as 50 percent of the body's muscle) will waste away through a process called selective atrophy.

Since fast-twitch fiber is the key muscle type responsible for increasing growth hormone, fast-twitch fiber must be the priority, particularly during middle age. Research by W. J. Evans at Tufts University demonstrates that adults, even to the age of 96, can respond to resistance training and experience strength and muscle gains of up to 200 percent, (*Exercise, nutrition, and aging*, 1992, Evans).

Older adults experience hormonal responses to exercise similar to their younger counterparts. However, it is extremely important for fast-twitch fiber to be maintained during aging by following a complete fitness plan that includes workouts targeted toward development of the three muscle fiber types.

For adults receiving growth hormone replacement therapy injections, unless prohibited, exercise should be included with their therapy. Researchers at the Department of Endocrinology at St. Bartholomew's Hospital in London conducted a study with 35 adults, average age 39, with GH deficiency and studied the impact of exercise with GH injections. The researchers show that future clinical trails involving GH should be have "planned exercise" as a part of the therapy, (*Effects of growth hormone replacement on physical performance and body composition in GH deficient adults*, 1999, Rodriguez-Arnao).

In study after study, researchers conclude that exercise increases GH release in young and old. Even to age 70 and beyond, high-intensity training increases GH.

Researchers placed perimenopausal women into three categories—active, relatively active, and inactive—to determine the impact of exercise on the symptoms of menopause. "Significant differences" in the symptoms of irritability, forgetfulness, headache, and other symptoms were reported between the inactive and the two active groups. (The relationship between physical activity and perimenopause," 1999, Li).

Additional information about exercise and aging:

Medline, A service of the National Library of Medical Science
Toll free: 888-346-3656
www.nlm.nih.gov/hinfo.html

National Institute on Aging
Toll free: 800-222-2225
www.nih.gov/nia

Comprehensive Training for Bodybuilders

The logic for a comprehensive, strategic fitness plan for anti-aging efforts also applies for people with the largest muscles in the world—bodybuilders. Many bodybuilders may only be exercising the slow-twitch muscle fiber with traditional forms of weightlifting that emphasize slow, squeezing repetitions. This means that the fast IIx fiber and perhaps the IIa muscle fiber, which may represent half of their muscle fiber, may be untouched during training.

A tremendous opportunity for bodybuilders lies in the creation of a training plan that develops all the body's muscle fiber. Bodybuilders implementing the Target Zone Training Method (Chapter 4), and working all the muscle fiber, might experience some extraordinary results. It would be helpful to hear results from bodybuilders who have used the Target Zone Training Method—E-mail your training experience and results to the publisher: pristine@charter.net.

Shock Muscle Memory

Personal trainers, bodybuilders, and athletes experienced in resistance training, understand muscle memory and the value of shocking muscles during workouts to pull out of a training plateau.

Researchers at the University of Canada investigated the effect of concurrent strength and endurance training on strength, endurance, endocrine hormone status, and muscle fiber. The findings from the 12-week study demonstrate that the combination of strength and endurance training yields a "significant increase in capillary development." And this research shows that "muscle memory" might be avoided with the combination of strength and endurance training, (*Effect of concurrent strength and endurance training on skeletal muscle properties and hormone concentrations in humans*, 2000, Bell).

"Intensive exercise . . . is associated with higher growth hormone and testosterone levels, and exercise may have a role in counteracting the decline in growth hormone with aging." (Relationship of physical exercise and aging to growth hormone production, 1999, Hurel, National Library of Medicine abstract).

Conclusion

Although all five major components of Synergy Fitness do not release growth hormone, all components are necessary. Significant improvements in health, fitness, and appearance can be made with a commitment to train only four to five hours a week, if done correctly.

The building blocks of your Strategic Fitness Plan are contained in the following chapters. The five major components of Synergy Fitness have a chapter each–ready to explain and fully illustrate exactly how to perform the exercises. These chapters will also serve as future reference guides for the various workouts contained in your fitness plan. Should you encounter problems on an exercise, simply refer back to the chapter and the illustrations.

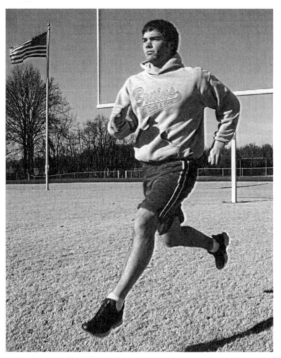

*Associated Press All-State high school football player
Jamie Richardson uses an advanced level of
Synergy Fitness to prepare for college football.*

6

Flexibility Fundamentals

Increasing Flexibility Makes You Feel Great!

Improving your flexibility will make you feel great . . . and look great! And it only takes 10 minutes, four times a week.

When it comes to flexibility, stretching is the name of the game. Stretching is not the type of exercise that will help you reach growth hormone release benchmarks, although newcomers to stretching frequently breathe and sweat heavily due to increased heart rate during the first few stretching sessions. Stretching clearly benefits the three types of muscle fibers by improving range of motion. Personally, I am a huge proponent of stretching. To emphasize the importance of this major component of Synergy Fitness, I frequently say that if I were forced to choose only one form of exercise, it would be stretching.

Researchers show that prolonged stretching (in the form of yoga) with moderate aerobic exercise and diet control will reduce cholesterol and significantly reverse hardening of the arteries (20 percent lesion regression) in adults with proven coronary atherosclerotic disease. After one year in a yoga program, research subjects lost weight, reduced cholesterol, and improved their exercise capacity, *(Retardation of coronary atherosclerosis with yoga lifestyle intervention, 2000, Manchanda).*

There were 21 adults in the yoga group and 21 in the control group that received conventional therapy (American Heart Association Step I Diet and Risk Factor Control). During the year, only one adult from the yoga group—verses eight from the diet control group—had bypass or angioplasty. Stretching may do much more than simply making you feel great by improving flexibility.

New Research Reverses the Rule on Stretching

Coaches have instilled it into the minds of their athletes as long as anyone can remember: stretch before you workout or play a game, the more the better. While I always stretch for 10 minutes prior to the Sprint 8 Workout for the warm-up benefit, new research totally reverses the pre-game philosophy of stretching.

Researchers show that athletes should not perform prolonged stretching routines before playing a game because it temporarily slows muscle activation.

Do not let this research be an excuse to not add the 10-Minute Stretching Routine (illustrated in this chapter) to your exercise plan. A full stretching program is important—just not an hour before the big game.

Getting Started

Stretching technique is everything! Since warming up prior to anaerobic training is an absolute rule never to be broken, this can be combined (multi-tasked) by using the 10-Minute Stretching Routine as your warm-up. This strategy is appropriate for the warm-up prior to training, but not before the game or a key practice session. The goal of the warm-up is to get the blood flowing and raise body temperature (one degree) prior to high-intensity workouts and athletic competition, and stretching does the job.

Improvement in flexibility produced by a consistent stretching routine has multiple joint-related benefits. New research shows that flexible hip flexors will prevent back pain. And strengthening abdominal muscles will help decrease back pain by providing additional support—so the lower back muscles do not have to carry the entire load.

My experience with stretching is that it is unlike any other form of exercise. The body seems to resist improved flexibility for the first 30 days or so. And this can be frustrating and cause you to want to quit. Be patient. It takes time to see real progress. Hang in there: the results are worth it! Just remember, you may not see improvement for 30 days. However, your patience will be rewarded because improved flexibility will make you feel great and it tones muscles (in just the right places).

"Prolonged" stretching decreases strength for up to an hour after stretching by slightly impairing muscle activation. (Reduced strength after passive stretch of the human plantar flexors, 2000, Fowles).

Physicians are called on to think about exercise for the aging population as a "medical prescription" that should include training for flexibility, strength, and endurance.
(Aging and Physical Activity, 2000, Leach).

Heads Up: Stretching Is Tough but Essential

Stretching can be . . . oh, heck . . . it's painful. There's no other way to say it; stretching hurts every time I perform the 10-Minute Stretching Routine. But in every case, when the routine is finished, I feel much better than when I started.

On days when I feel really stiff (in other words, most days), I have a motivational cue that I silently say to myself: "get tough... and get focused," and I move into the (not-so-comfortable) hold position. When my mind begins to play tricks on me about why I can afford to skip stretching today, I immediately quit thinking, move into the start position, take a deep breath, and say to myself silently, *"Ready, Set, GO!"* and pull down to the hold position for 30 seconds. I use this self-motivation cue with all forms of training.

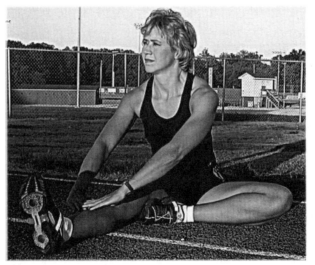

Photographs by Kathy Campbell

Certified personal trainer and triathlete, Melanie Joyner, begins the 10-Minute Stretching Routine as a warm-up prior to running.

The 10-Minute Stretching Routine

The stretching routine illustrated in this chapter is recommended for all ages and fitness levels. The 10-Minute Stretching Routine (10 minutes three to five days per week) is programmed into every Strategic Fitness Plan in this book—typically for four days a week. And this stretching routine should be performed more frequently than other forms of training that require varying recovery periods.

Research in Copenhagen demonstrates that a "single stretch hold" can increase muscle "elastic relaxation" by 30 percent for an hour after stretching. And long-term stretching increases joint range of motion, (*Passive properties of human skeletal muscle during stretch maneuvers*, 1998, Magnusson).

All stretching positions in the prescribed routine are static, which means no bouncing. Slowly move into the illustrated stretching position and get "fully stretched." You will know when you are fully stretched when you "feel the limit" (cannot go any further). Again, as you begin your stretching routine, **DO NOT BOUNCE.** This can cause injury. Move in "slow motion."

You should feel slight discomfort but no sharp pain. Hold the position for 30 seconds (without bouncing) then, very slowly, ease out of the position before going to the next stretching position.

The stretching positions in the 10-Minute Stretching Routine impact most major muscle groups, except chest, shoulders, and upper back. For time saving through multi-tasking exercises, upper body stretching is programmed to perform during weight training.

Flexibility is dependent on the "duration" of stretching position, and the best "stretch hold" is 30 seconds. (The effect of time on static stretch on the flexibility of the hamstring muscles, 1994, Bandy).

1. Hamstring Stretch

Sitting on the floor with one leg extended and the other leg bent, slowly pull forward. You will feel the target area—hamstrings and lower back.

Once in the fully stretched position (there should be slight discomfort, but no pain), hold for 30 seconds. Then, slowly, ease out of the position. On cold days, or days when you feel less flexible, you may want to repeat the 30 second hold position before switching legs.

Almost every muscle group receives benefit from this stretching position—hamstrings, calves, Achilles tendons, groin, quadriceps (quads), obliques, shoulders, upper and lower back. This is a core stretching position and serves as a warm-up for the other stretching positions.

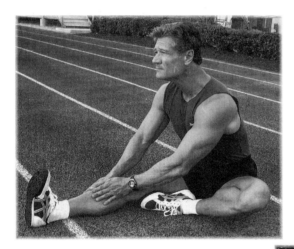

Start

Photographs by Holly Campbell

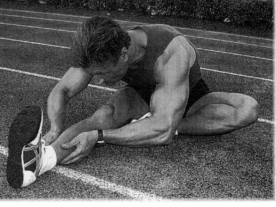

Pull forward position

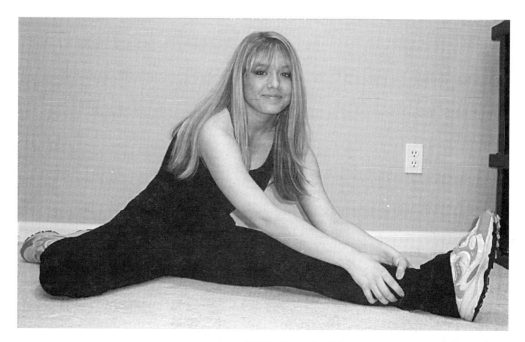

Holly Campbell demonstrates the hurdle stretch.
Stretching is great exercise for teenagers.

Stretching is recommended for healthy adults of all ages, teens and children.

2. Hurdle Stretch

There are four parts to this exercise. Keeping one leg in the extended position, bring the other leg to the side in a bent position making an *L* shape with your legs, slowly pull forward to the extended leg and hold for 30 seconds. There should be discomfort, but no sharp pain in the fully stretched pull forward position.

Start

Pull forward position

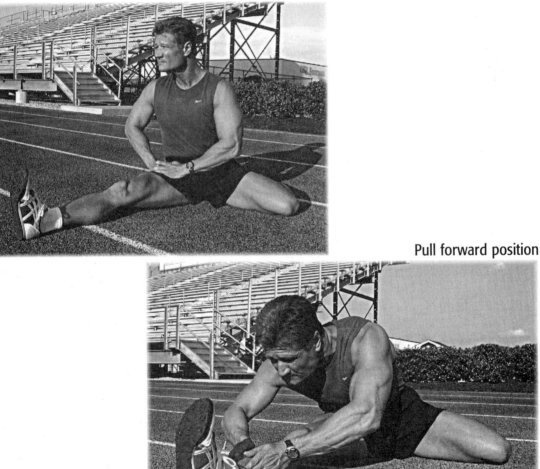

Without moving your legs, lie back on the floor, as shown in the third photo. This will stretch a different set of muscles—quads, knees, ankles, lower back and the hip flexors receive maximum benefit from this stretching position. Then, sit up slowly and pull forward a second time. Once in the fully stretched position, hold for 30 seconds. Then repeat on the other side.

Lay back position

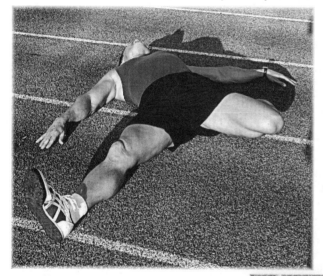

**Repeat
pull forward position**

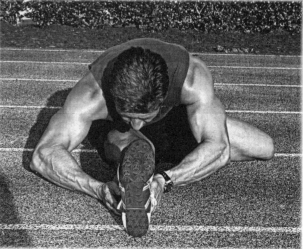

3. Hamstring Leg-Raise Stretch

The hamstring leg-raise stretch is a difficult stretching position. Lying on your back, raise one leg and grab your ankle. Hold for 30 seconds in the fully stretched position.

Unless you have been stretching regularly, you may need to grab your sock or your pant leg. Repeat with the other leg.

Doing these stretching exercises will begin to increase your range of motion, and flexibility gains should be noticeable after six weeks.

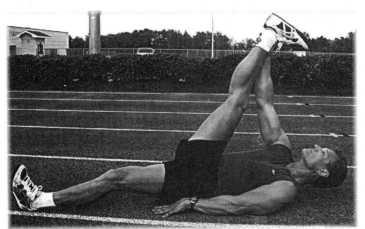

Leg raise

Leg tucked position

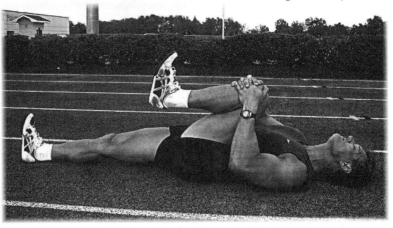

10-Minute Stretching Routine

#1 Hamstring stretch

#2 Hurdle stretch

#3 Hamstring leg raise stretch

#4 Split-leg stretch

#5 Calf stretch

Note:
Stretching is unlike any other form
of exercise that provides positive
results quickly. Your body seems
to fight flexibility for the first
few weeks. Then, between four to six
weeks, your body stops resisting and
agrees to increase flexibility.

4. Split-Legs Stretch

There are four parts to this stretching position. Start: sit on the floor and spread your legs as illustrated in the first photo. If you are new to flexibility training, hold in the starting position for 30 seconds.

Start position

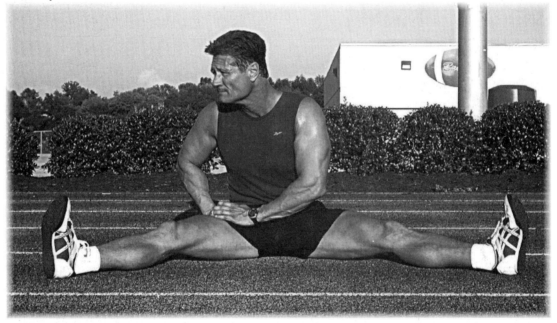

Next, move slowly into the "pull right" position. Keep your legs straight, and very slowly pull your body toward the right foot. Hold for 30 seconds. Then, pull your body to the left leg for the 30 second hold position, keeping your legs straight.

Pull right position

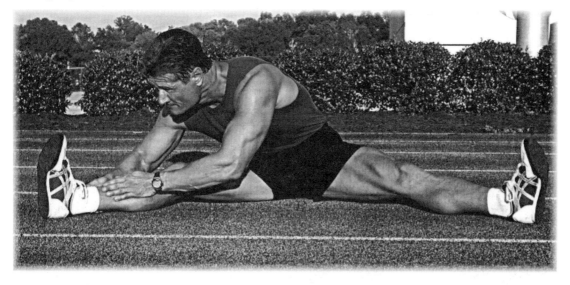

For the final stretching position, pull down to the center for a 30 second hold in the fully stretched position as shown.

Center

Photographs by Kathy Campbell

5. Calf Stretch

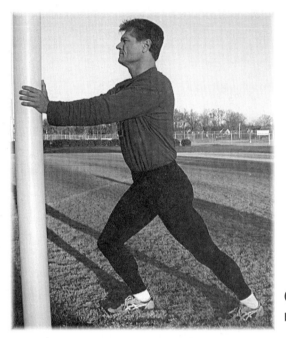

Calf stretch position, no bouncing

Reverse legs and fully stretch achilles tendon

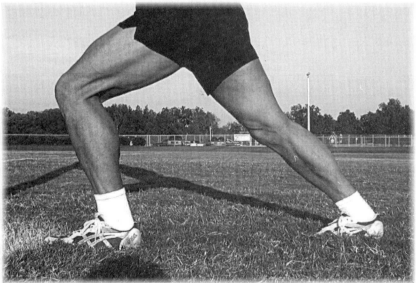

Optional Stretching Positions

Hamstring Stretching

Hamstrings, calves, ankles, and lower back benefit from the following stretching positions. In the bent split-legs stretching position demonstrated by personal trainer Bambi LaFont, RN, (age 41, and mother of two) slightly turn toes inward to stretch the outer calves and ankles.

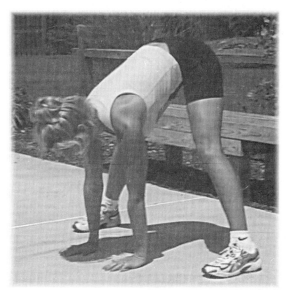

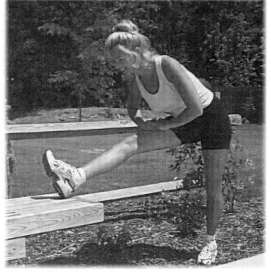

Slightly press down to stretch hamstring

Side Torso Stretch

Stretching sides in this position targets the upper body trunk, abs, ribcage and upper back. Move into this position and hold for 30 seconds on both sides as shown by Kristi McCarver and Shay Ingram.

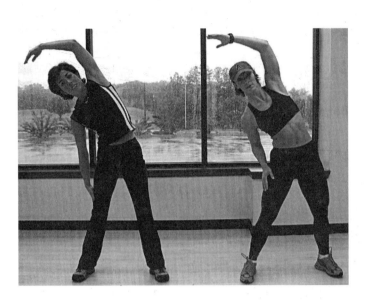

Butterfly Stretch

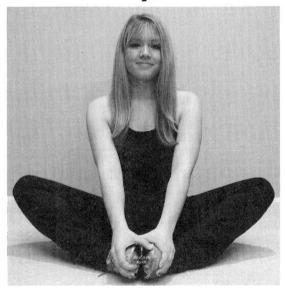

Lower Back

The basic lower-back stretching position is performed by IFPA certified personal trainer, Melanie Joyner, JD, (age 36, mother of three). Lying facedown, place hands under shoulders to start. Slowly press upward. As you "feel the limit"in your lower back, stop and hold for 30 seconds.

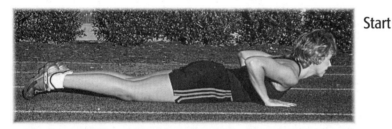

Start

Beginning level up position (below)

Front view

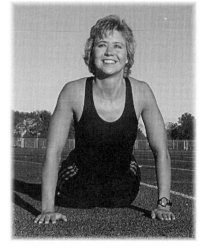

Advanced up position (above)

Stretching for Children

Recent research shows that stretching can prevent injury in children. Researchers conclude that there is a strong association between decreased flexibility and ankle injury in children, (*Limited dorsiflexion predisposes to injuries of the ankle in children*, 2000, Tabritzi). Children can easily perform the 10-Minute Stretching Routine.

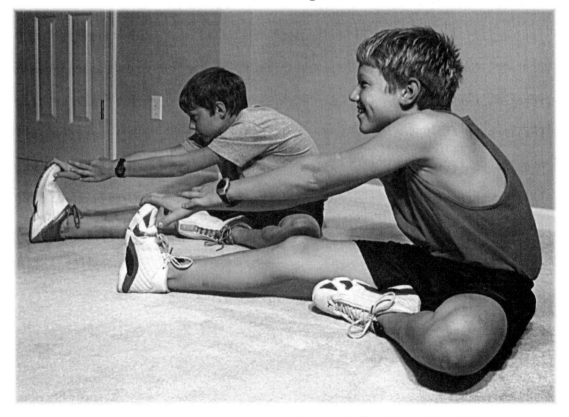

John Campbell and Scott Metcalf demonstrate the first stretching position of 10-Minute Stretching Routine.

Upper Body Flexibility

Upper body stretching may be performed with the 10-Minute Stretching Routine, independently, or the Synergy Fitness way and save time by multi-tasking upper body flexibility training with resistance training.

During the 1-minute recovery between weightlifting sets, simply take 30 seconds to stretch one side of the upper body. Repeat for the other side during a following set.

NOTE: Upper Body Flexibility Training

To save time–multi-task exercises by stretching the body part being worked between sets during weight training

---

Stretch the body part being worked—it's a good rule to follow during weight training. Just like in the 10-Minute Stretching Routine, slowly move to the "fully stretched position" and hold for 30 seconds. Do not bounce during stretching in order to maximize results and reduce risk of injury. Once in the fully stretched position, "feel the limit" and the slight discomfort (at the limit), hold for 30 seconds, and slowly ease out of the position.

Even at advanced levels of fitness, adding stretching to weight training can cause initial soreness, and even injury. As with any new exercise addition, gradually add "flexibility fundamentals" into your resistance training. And remember, no fast movements. Pretend you are moving in slow motion as you move into and out of stretching positions.

The following photographs show methods of stretching the major upper body muscle groups—chest, shoulders, and upper back.

Upper Back Stretching

The hammer throw stretching position resembles the Olympic event. Grab a stationary bar as illustrated. Lean backward to fully stretch the upper back (lat) muscles. Lean slightly to the left (fully stretching the left lat muscle), and hold 30 seconds. Repeat, leaning to the right. Perform this while working your upper back during weightlifting.

Hammer throw stretching position

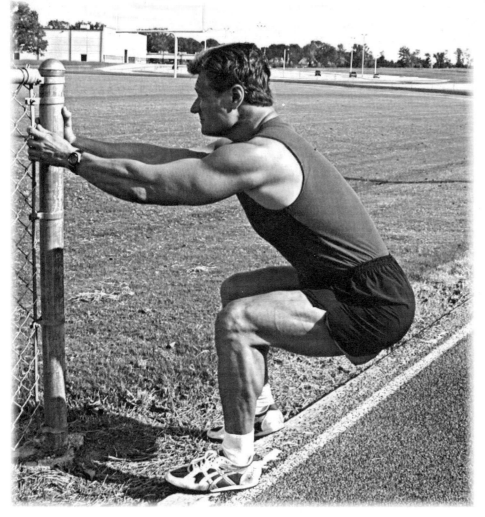

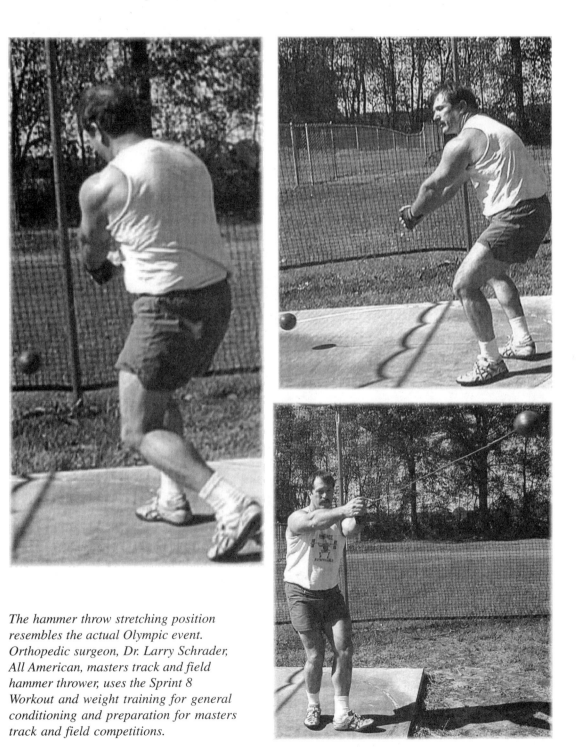

The hammer throw stretching position resembles the actual Olympic event. Orthopedic surgeon, Dr. Larry Schrader, All American, masters track and field hammer thrower, uses the Sprint 8 Workout and weight training for general conditioning and preparation for masters track and field competitions.

Chest Stretching

The javelin chest stretching position shown in the illustration is very effective in stretching the chest muscles. This stretching position is similar to the position you assume before throwing a javelin—palm up, extended arm.

Use the javelin chest stretching position while working your chest. Keep the arm stationary and extended, *palm up*, back straight, and chest out. Once in this position, lean forward and "feel the limit" in your chest. Hold for 30 seconds. Repeat on the other side.

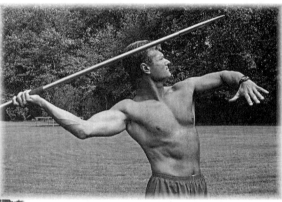

Javelin stretching position

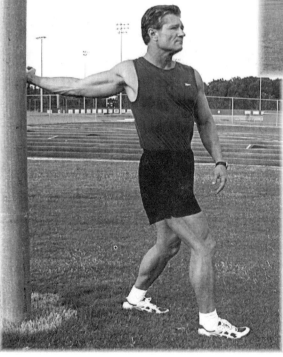

Keeping your palm up (just like throwing the javelin) moves the target area to the chest.

Shoulder Stretching

The discus shoulder stretching position resembles the shoulder movement of throwing a discus. Hold a stationary bar *(palm down),* with your body upright and chest out, lean forward, and fully stretch the shoulder. Hold for 30 seconds. Repeat on the other side. Perform this stretch when working shoulders.

Discus stretching position

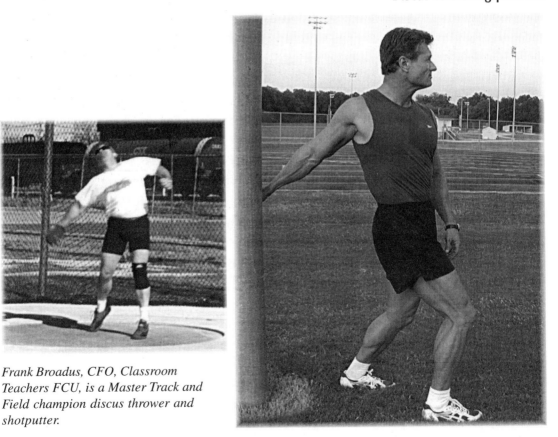

Frank Broadus, CFO, Classroom Teachers FCU, is a Master Track and Field champion discus thrower and shotputter.

Conclusion

Stretching is a major component of total fitness. It has numerous health benefits in addition to the joint/ligament benefits of increasing flexibility. The 10-Minute Stretching Routine is designed for all ages and levels of conditioning. This routine is programmed into all Strategic Fitness Plans (Chapter 11).

The next chapter discusses endurance training. Experienced long distance runners know, and research proves, endurance-trained athletes have greater muscle tightness and need extra flexibility training, (*Lower extremity muscular flexibility in long distance runners*, 1993, Wang)

Applying the concepts in "Flexibility Fundamentals" is important for everyone, but particularly for endurance-trained athletes, such as distance swimmers, 10K runners, and marathon runners, as well as adults wanting to increase their fitness training capability.

Keep your book open, and try the 10-Minute Stretching Routine today. Stretching will make you feel great and tone your muscles in just the right places! Remember—flexibility training is unlike other forms of fitness training where you typically experience quick results. It may take several weeks before you see improvement in flexibility. Hang in there. Positive results will come with persistence.

Stretching can be somewhat painful initially, so when your mind starts playing games about passing on the stretching routine, just say to yourself, "Ready, Set, GO!" and start the routine.

7

Energizing Endurance

Building Your Endurance Base

Cardio workouts build endurance. And the endurance base is necessary for all other fitness components. Endurance is typically the measurement used for general fitness.

Although most sports qualify as anaerobic exercise, the aerobic base for athletic performance and fitness improvement is vitally important. Performance in any sport or fitness plan that includes anaerobic sprinting or running intervals lasting over eight seconds has an aerobic component supplying oxygen to the body.

Don't let the term *sprinting* frighten you. Sprinting, and other forms of high-intensity exercise, can be performed in many ways. Sprinting does not necessarily mean running at full speed (for details, see Chapter 8).

Aerobic processes contribute up to 40 percent of the energy used during the first 30 seconds of high-intensity exercise.
(Relative importance of aerobic an anaerobic energy release during short-lasting exhausting bicycle exercise, 1989, Medbo).

Cardio Training

The goal for cardio training is to achieve the aerobic target heart rate (age specific) and maintain that rate for 20 to 30 minutes.

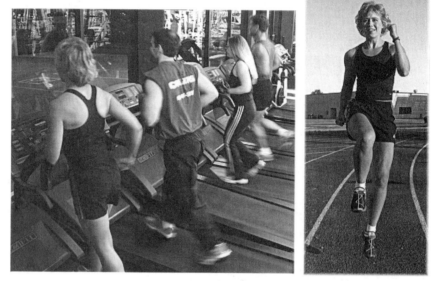

Cardio workouts can be performed by adults of all ages: aerobic bench-step classes; at the gym on a bike, stepper, rowing machine, elliptical trainer, treadmill; and outside jogging, cycling, power walking, hiking, cross-country skiing, swimming, etc.

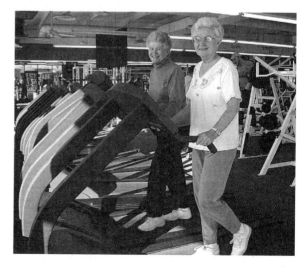

Wilma Diffee & Joan Vidrine on treadmills.

Figuring Your Target Heart Rate for Cardio Training

The typical formula used to calculate aerobic target heart rate is 220 – your age = maximum heart rate. The target range becomes the maximum heart rate x 65 to 85 percent for fit adults.

For beginners, the rate should begin at the 50 percent point and slowly build to 70 percent. The 50 percent target can be easily achieved through power walking (fast walking).

The aerobic target heart rate calculation for age 50:

220 – 50 = 170 max heart rate (HR)
170 x .65 = 110 lower aerobic HR
170 x .85 = 145 highest HR

The aerobic target heart rate range for a 50-year-old is between 110 and 145 with the average being 127 heartbeats per minute. During cardio workouts, the goal is to maintain an exercising heart rate of 127 and sustain it for a 20 to 30 minute session. This is a great way to burn calories and build an aerobic base for high-intensity, GH-releasing exercise.

Making Cardio Fun

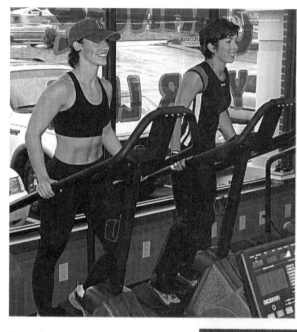

Shay Ingram and Kristi McCarver using steppers at the gym.

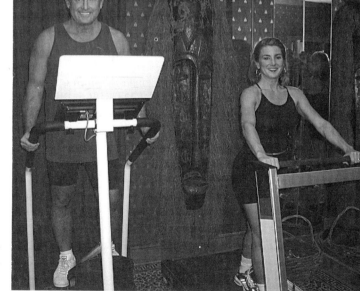

Dr. Bob and Tabitha Souder working out in their home gym.

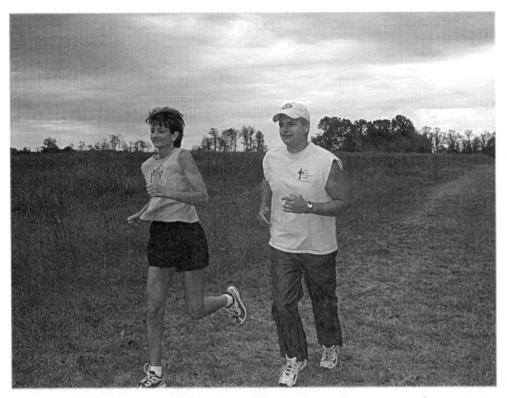

Jon and Susan Parrish, owners of Lord's Gym in Jackson, Tennessee, getting in cardio by jogging together on a cross-country course.

Aerobic vs. Anaerobic Training

The debate of aerobic exercise verses anaerobic training is short-sighted and misses the theme of this book. It is not a question of one over the other. These two forms of training are interrelated and are both vital components of Synergy Fitness.

Researchers show that the health profile and total body fitness for women can be improved dramatically with aerobics and resistance training. (Resistance training combined with bench-step aerobics enhances women's health profile, 2001, Kraemer).

Research demonstrates "significant differences" in the release of growth hormone by anaerobic and aerobic exercise. Anaerobic training clearly achieves GH release. (Effect of anaerobic and aerobic exercise of equal duration and work on plasma growth hormone levels, 1984, Vanhelder).

When it comes to increasing growth hormone, anaerobic exercise increases GH significantly higher than aerobic. However, remember this point. The endurance base—built by aerobic exercise—makes anaerobic exercise possible. These two forms of training are interrelated and are both vital components of Synergy Fitness.

Does cardio training increase GH? Yes, but it may take two training sessions during the same day. If you are *not* a time-crunched adult and have plenty of time, you can certainly try this. Researchers show that a second exercise session during the same day will increase growth hormone, (*Increased neuroendocrine response to a repeated bout of endurance exercise*, 2001, Ronsen).

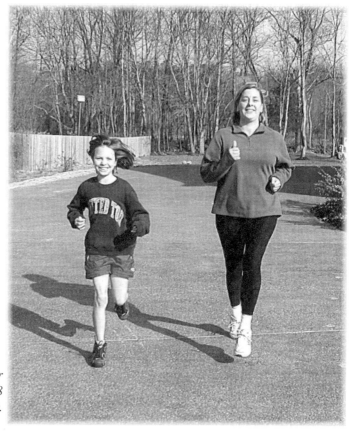

Cindy and Halie Miller, mother and daughter, doing the Sprint 8 Workout in their driveway.

Time Crunch Tip:
Multi-Task Endurance Exercise With Anaerobic Training

Accomplishing both aerobic and anaerobic training simultaneously may be achieved by multi-tasking exercises in your fitness plan. Sprinting, bleacher running, and plyometric drills achieve anaerobic training goals. And the brief walk-back to the start (1.5 to 2 minutes maximum) will keep the heart rate over aerobic target heart rate for approximately 20-minutes.

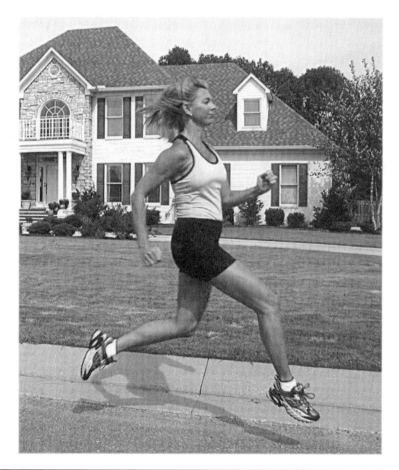

Bleacher Running Multi-Tasks Anaerobic and Aerobic Fitness Training

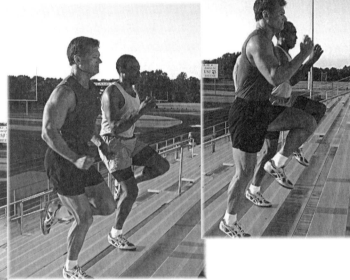

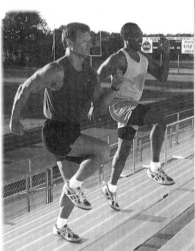

Running bleachers with my running partner,
Nate Robertson, State Games
100 and 200 meters 2001 champion (age 50).

Photographs by Kathy Campbell

Impact of Anaerobic Sprints on Heart Rate

The following graph illustrates the impact of the Sprint 8 Workout on heart rate. During the sprint, the heart rate rises far above the aerobic target heart rate. And even during the 1.5 to 2 minute walk-back to the starting line, even during the recovery period, the aerobic target heart rate is achieved. The cardiac target rate is maintained during the entire Sprint 8 Workout.

For middle-aged adults and older, heart rate monitors are available and inexpensive compared to their fitness improvement value ($50 to $120). I use the POLAR brand and check my heart rate monthly for changes in aerobic performance, (www.polarusa.com or 800-227-1314).

Impact of anaerobic sprints on heart rate

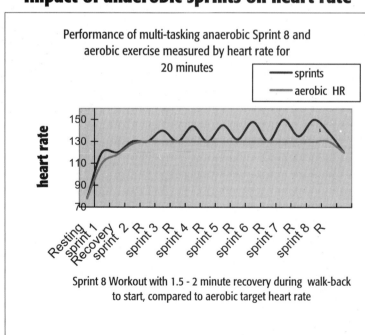

Performance of multi-tasking anaerobic Sprint 8 and aerobic exercise measured by heart rate for 20 minutes

Sprint 8 Workout with 1.5 - 2 minute recovery during walk-back to start, compared to aerobic target heart rate

Heart monitor kits include two items—a wristwatch-type heart rate monitor and a strap that fits around the chest at the ribcage level. The strap measures your heartbeats per minute and sends the reading to your wristwatch monitor. There are no dangling wires to struggle with while you walk or jog. For the beginner, this is an extra safety feature.

Interval Training

Interval training is discussed in *Accelerating with Anaerobics* (Chapter 8) with over-speed training programs designed to reduce running time per mile. Running intervals will improve speed and endurance. And it is possible for triathletes, marathon, and mid-distance runners to reduce their running times significantly with interval training and sprinting.

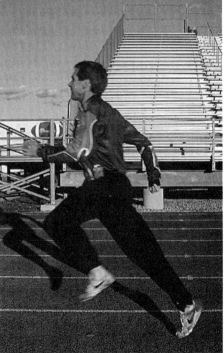

Leon Hoover uses the Sprint 8 Workout to increase speed and endurance.

Got Shoes?
Caution: Road Running May Cause Orthopedic Problems

Long distance (street) runners need to replace running shoes much more frequently than you may expect. Mileage, body weight, and running surfaces cause wear on running shoes. Typically, every three months (and less for some runners) it is time to get new shoes. Street running requires shoes with maximum padding.

Don't be stingy on running shoes. Running is not an expensive sport. So what if you spend 25 cents a mile on shoes if it prevents permanent damage to your knees, hips, and lower back. You may save thousands of dollars in future healthcare bills.

Stress fractures may develop while running. This is a significant problem for long distance runners, (*Interventions for preventing and treating stress fractures and stress reactions of bones of the lower limbs in young adults*, 2000, Gillespie).

Researchers show that absorbing insoles can reduce the risk of stress fractures, and that additional calcium nutrition is helpful in preventing injury to the bone. And a pneumatic knee brace during treatment of a stress fracture (caused by running) will significantly reduce the healing time to recommence training.

I have found that running distance on the street causes me to have bone problems. The constant pounding hurts my lower back. Distance running is associated with bone problems, while intervals and sprinting are associated with increased muscle pulls (without adequate flexibility, strength, and warm-up before training). Hamstrings are the likely targets.

Ask any orthopedic surgeon about the long-term impact of pounding the pavement, and you will hear that you should not run on the street. I have never experienced any problems running on a good track. Also, aerobic machines like bikes and treadmills (with a flexible landing area) seem to minimize these problems.

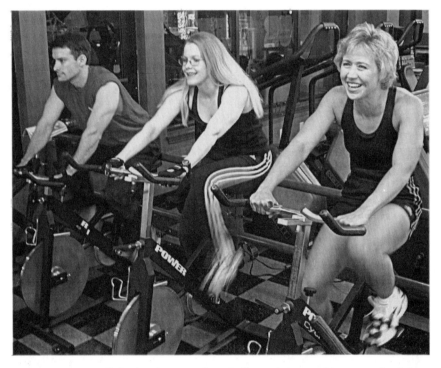

Spinning is great for cardio training and easy on the joints.
Matt & Melissa Marvin, Melanie Joyner.

Endurance Building Supplements

Aerobic muscular endurance can be increased with protein supplements combined with aerobic and resistance training. The need for additional protein is clear in recent research. Energy drinks in the future will all contain protein along with vitamins, minerals, electrolytes, etc. Remember: 25 grams of protein after training is recommended (Chapter 1).

Researchers report that six weeks of amino-acid supplements increased endurance for women untrained in aerobics and weight training. (Effects of exercise training and amino-acid supplementation on body composition and physical performance in untrained women, 2001, Antonio).

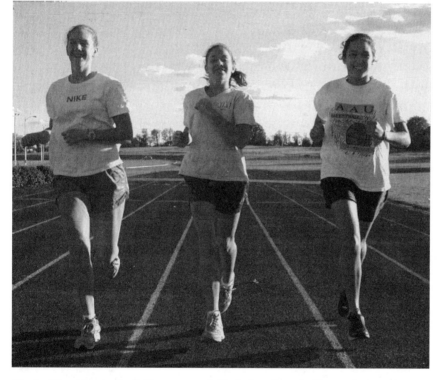

Kacie Fite, Carrie Beth Henson, and Christine Campbell running on the track in off-season training for basketball.

Researchers at the University of Maryland show that strength training improves endurance. *(Effects of strength training on lactate thresholds and endurance performance,* 1991, Marcinik).

Conclusion

The endurance base is very important. The Strategic Fitness Plans in Chapter 11 contain workouts called "Cardio-20" and "Cardio-30" (20 or 30 minutes) for aerobic endurance building training.

The workouts in the Strategic Fitness Plans will also develop an endurance base (if the exercises are "multi-tasked" appropriately). For example, during the Sprint 8 Workout, if you limit recovery (during the walk-back to the start) to less than 1.5 to 2 minutes, you will achieve 20 minutes of endurance training simultaneously with the anaerobic workout. And weightlifting, in a multi-tasked format, will build your endurance base. Limit the recovery between sets to 1.5 to 2 minutes, and you will build the endurance base in addition to building strength.

The "missing ingredient" in many fitness plans—anaerobic training—will be discussed in the following chapter.

8

Accelerating Growth Hormone Release with Anaerobics

Anaerobic workouts improve athletic performance and accelerate the release of synergistic growth hormone like no other form of fitness training. Research clearly demonstrates that anaerobic training, by far, has the greatest potential for significantly increasing your body's natural release of growth hormone (GH). Yet it is often missing in many fitness plans.

To develop a sprinter's physique, it will be necessary to build and increase your IIx super fast muscle fiber. The average person has 10 percent of the super fast IIx muscle fiber, aerobic trained athletes have 5 percent IIx fiber, and sprint trained athletes have 40 percent IIx. See **Muscle Fiber Composition** on page 92 in Chapter 4 for details.

You build by doing, so the goal needs to be a balanced approach targeting slow twitch, fast IIa and Super fast IIx muscle during your training.

Anaerobic Workouts Need No Special Equipment

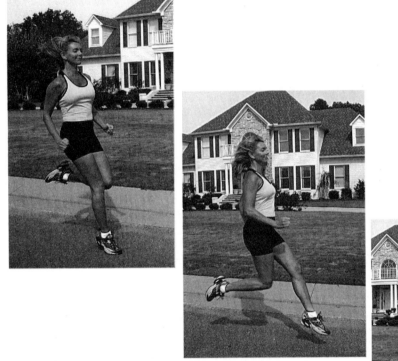

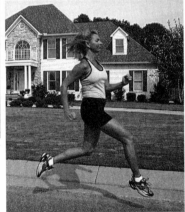

AFAA Certified Personal Trainer, Bambi LaFont, BS, RN, age 41, performs the Sprint 8 Workout at home.

Photographs by Kathy Campbell

Sprint-trained athletes can increase growth hormone levels to 10 times the normal level, say researchers at Loughborough University, England. And there is an 82 percent difference between sprint training and endurance training in the ability to produce GH. This is due to "peak power output and peak blood lactate response to the sprint." In fitness training, only an intense, anaerobic workout can produce a significant increase in growth hormone, (*Growth hormone responses to treadmill sprinting in sprint- and endurance-trained athletes*, 1996, Nevill).

Comparing the ability of different types of exercise to produce growth hormone release, anaerobic training receives the highest marks from medical researchers. (Hormonal and metabolic response to three types of exercise of equal duration and external work output, 1985, Vanhelder).

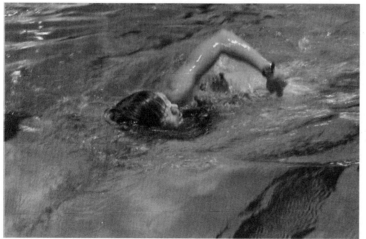

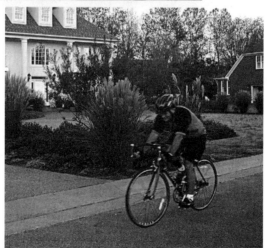

Chris LaFont cycling.

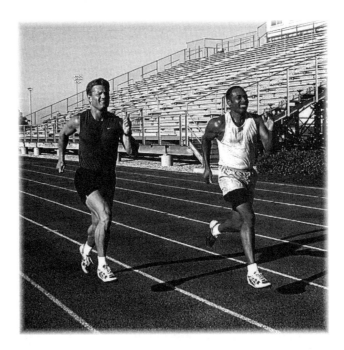

Running warm-up sprints with my main running partner, Nate Robertson, age 50. Nate is the 2001 State Senior Olympic Games 100-meters and 200-meters champion.

Whether you use the Sprint 8 Workout with running, swimming, cycling, power walking up an incline, or a different method, anaerobic training is absolutely necessary in a comprehensive strategic fitness plan. I wish I could tell you the Sprint 8 Workout only takes 20 minutes and will get you in great physical condition, easily, and cover a multitude of dietary sins. I cannot. However, I *can* tell you that the Sprint 8 Workout will get you in great physical condition, only takes 20 minutes, and can cover some "off diet" fast food meals. But this workout is tough.

Don't let the word *sprint* frighten you. The Sprint 8 Workout doesn't necessarily mean running at full speed. If you are 70, you'll need eight repetitions of some type of anaerobic exercise lasting 10 to 30 seconds, with 1 to 2 minutes of recovery in between. This may be accomplished by sprint or power walking past two or three mailboxes in front of your home. The key is for you to hit all four GH-release benchmarks—out-of-breath, body temperature increase, lactic acid, and adrenal response (see Chapter 1).

If you are 17 and in shape, an athlete, or middle-aged and fit, then the intensity of your Sprint 8 Workouts will need to be at a high level to achieve GH-release benchmarks. The intensity of the Sprint 8 Workout is relative to age, fitness status, and training experience.

The Sprint 8 Workout

The running version of the Sprint 8 Workout will reach all GH-release benchmarks in one 20 minute session. Researchers suggest that 20 minutes of exercise at 90 percent intensity may serve as a suitable test for GH secretion, (Sutton, 1976). The Sprint 8 Workout is a powerful tool in any fitness plan to increase growth hormone naturally.

Sprint swimming, peddling, stepping, and uphill walking may accomplish the same GH-release objectives; however, the running version does not require a pool, a hill, or any special equipment. You do not need a track, although a track is more comfortable and safer than the streets. Actually, all you need is a sidewalk and markers (mailboxes work great) approximately 70-yards apart.

Aerobic gym units and some treadmills offer high-intensity programs that allow you to run, peddle, and step at a high rate for 15 to 30 seconds and more—with light recovery periods in between. And this may also achieve GH-release benchmarks. Just remember—all four GH-release benchmarks need to be reached during your workout.

The Sprint 8 Workout is running eight repetitions of progressive (build-up) sprints. Each sprint should last for 8 to 12 seconds. Most people can cover approximately 60-meters or 70-yards in 8 to 12 seconds.

For the fit individual, the first sprint should actually start at a jogging pace (approximately 30 percent speed/intensity) and progressively build to 50 percent speed/intensity.

After crossing the finish mark (mailbox, yard line, etc), gradually slow down. To avoid common "stop/start" hamstring injuries, take a full 10-yards to slow to a stop after running the full 70-yards. Turn, and take 1.5 to 2 minutes to walk back to the start. The walk-back serves as an important recovery period before the next sprint that will enable you to exert more intensity into the following sprint.

The gradual slow-down at the end of the sprint is extremely important. Injuries occur most frequently during starting and stopping. Ease into the start, and ease off the sprint after crossing the finish line. This means you should have covered approximately 10 to 20-yards beyond the finish during the slowing process. Again, make sure you have your physician's approval before beginning, take plenty of fluids, and slowly build to this program.

The second sprint repetition will begin at a 40 percent pace and progressively increase intensity to 60 percent speed/intensity. Likewise, the third sprint starts at a 50 percent pace and builds to 70 percent intensity. The first day, stop at the fourth sprint unless you are sprint-conditioned.

Slowly add one or two sprints to your workout every session until you get to the full eight sprints. Once you are sprint-conditioned, the last three to four sprints should be at 90-95 percent speed/intensity—this will reach all GH-release benchmarks. When you are out of breath and your muscles are slightly burning, you will know you have reached the GH-release benchmarks.

WARNING!

Sprinting in heat can be dangerous!

Since 1953, over one hundred football players have died on the field. An expert who appeared on the television show *Real Sports* to discuss the death of a pro-football player during summer camp and the death of a 5'10" 280 pound high-school football player who died while practicing in the hot sun for six hours, provided insightful information. The deaths, he said, were caused by "a malfunction of the heat regulation system in the brain." The combination of extreme heat, heavy clothing, lack of fluids, and sprint-type anaerobic sports like football, can become dangerous.

Drinking water between every sprint is my own practice on hot days in the summer sun. Anaerobic training is demanding, and it increases body temperature quickly. Medical research in 2001 shows that growth hormone release will be significantly decreased without adequate fluid, (Peyreign, 2001). Common sense with anaerobic training is a must. And when in doubt about any aspect of fitness training, contact your physician.

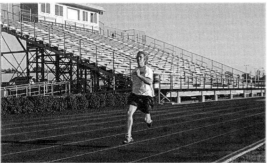

Adam Simon (left) and Trell Shivley (right) use the Sprint 8 Workout for high school soccer off-season training.

Sprint 8 Workout

Progressive Anaerobic Sprints

1st Sprint	Begin jogging; build to **50%** speed/intensity. Walk-back recovery (1.5 to 2 minutes)
2nd Sprint	Begin 40% pace, build to **60%**
3rd Sprint	Begin 50%, build to **70%**
4th Sprint	Begin 60%, build to **80%**
5th Sprint	Begin 70%, build to **90%**
6th Sprint	Build to **95%**
7th Sprint	**95%**
8th Sprint	**95%**
Cool-down	Walk or jog 2 minutes

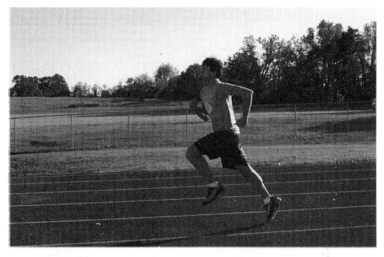

Whether you are 17 or 70, exercise intensity is relative by age and conditioning. Your anaerobic program should be fun, fast, and very effective—at any age. However, keep in mind that the Sprint 8 Workout is very demanding and could be hazardous to your health without a slow, preconditioning, build-up period and a physical exam by your physician.

Start with two to four progressive sprints the first day, and make them easy. Progressively build by adding one or two sprint repetitions during future workouts.

Warning for Ex Jocks

Many former athletes implementing the Sprint 8 Workout begin feeling so good during the first two to three weeks that they decide to see just how fast they can run on the last sprint.

A few have pulled hamstrings. The reason is that their slow-twitch muscles have been maintained through the years and feel good, but without realizing it, their fast-twitch muscles have atrophied and decreased in strength, size, and flexibility.

Don't be misled by the feeling of your strong slow-twitch muscles; it will take several months of strengthening the fast-twitch muscles before you can push the intensity levels beyond 70 to 80 percent speed.

Expect some soreness after the first few anaerobic workouts. Even for the young and fit, sprinting works muscles not touched by most exercises. Anaerobic exercise requires more warm-up time and a progressive conditioning period. Be wise—gradually build to the Sprint 8 Workout.

Expect for it to be difficult to perform anaerobic training some days. On these days, I say to myself, "Ready, Set, GO…make the effort." Even when I do not feel like training, saying "Ready, Set, GO," is my personal cue to "get tough" on myself, get focused, start, and finish the program.

Sprinting on a Treadmill?

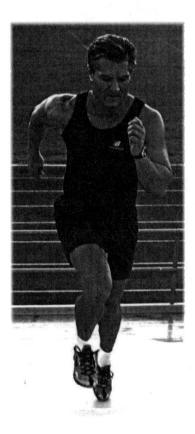

Dr. Randall Bush wanted the benefit of the growth hormone increasing Sprint 8 Workout, but he needed to stay indoors. His solution was to discover a way to make the program work on a treadmill. And he did.

Out-of-the-box thinking led Dr. Bush to experiment with treadmill intensity levels by raising the running platform five degrees in elevation. Since some treadmills take time to build speed, Dr. Bush (right) increases his sprint speed to 8 mph and does not begin to count the sprint time of 10 seconds until the treadmill achieves the 8 mph speed. It can take 10 seconds or more to build to this speed.

Once he achieves the 10 seconds of sprinting, he immediately punches in a 1.8 mph speed to serve as the walk-back during recovery. While this method may sound somewhat awkward, Dr. Bush has found a viable way of performing the Sprint 8 Workout on a treadmill.

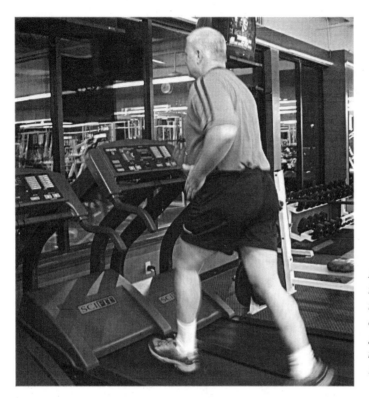

Dr. Randall Bush performs the Sprint 8 Workout on a treadmill by increasing the elevation to a 5 percent grade, running sprints at 8 mph, and walking during recovery at 1.8 mph.

Training Intensity (Not Training Volume) Determines Athletic Performance Improvement

A common mistake made by athletes during the off-season is designing a fitness plan to improve performance based on the strategy "more is better." The attitude seems to be, "I need to run more or lift more during the off season." This strategy will inspire an incorrectly designed fitness plan. It is human to think more training is better, but over training can harm your body.

In a training slump? Researchers show that "training intensity," not "training volume" is the key factor in performance improvement, *(Effects of training on performance in competitive swimming,* 1995, Mujika). You may want to rethink the strategy of "more training volume," report researchers investigating methods to improve the performance of athletes who are in a slump, *(Responses to training in cross-country skiers, 1999,* Gaskill). Better strategy—step-up the intensity of your training.

Improving Speed Endurance

Speed endurance is a term used to describe the endurance demands for most sports. It is developed by multi-tasking sprint work with progressively shorter recovery times. The proven training method is to run sprints at 95 to 100 percent speed/intensity and progressively decrease the recovery walk-back time between sprints, beginning at 2 minutes.

If you are a high school athlete, you may need to begin at Fitness Level Four prescribed in the Strategic Fitness Plans. Off-season college and professional athletes begin at Level Five—the Sprint 8 Workout followed by 4 x 150 meter sprints at 95 percent speed/intensity.

The goal of speed endurance training is to increase aerobic and anaerobic capacity that is required by sports with **repetitive bursts of speed**—football, soccer, basketball, baseball, tennis, boxing, karate, and others. "Speed endurance" development and "speed" development are two separate forms of training.

Improving Speed

Despite popular belief, running speed is not simply a genetic issue. Speed is a skill. And skills may be improved—with the correct information and training. Developing speed takes specific training knowledge and good resources are available. I have my own favorite book, video and E-mail newsletter to recommend.

Sports Speed, by Dintiman, Ward and Tellez (Tom Tellez coached Olympian Carl Lewis), is an excellent book specifically aimed at improving all aspects of speed. If you are a high school or college athlete involved in a sport where speed is important, you need the information in this book, www.humankinetics.com.

Speed Dynamics is the best video series I have seen on speed development. The three tape series features two nationally recognized track coaches, Kevin O'Donnell and Loren Seagrave.

Ross Dunton of Dunton Sports Management produces a quality speed development email newsletter. The daily E-mail newsletter is inexpensive and full of information, www.coachr.org/tandfnews.htm.

Do not allow the quest for the endurance aspect of "speed endurance" to overshadow the speed work. To build speed, take the full recovery (during the walk-back between sprints) so you have adequate energy for speed technique improvement and power development during training.

Over-Speed Training

Over-speed training is running at a faster pace than you are capable. This is possible by running downhill or with some type of speed-assisted device. Interval training for marathoners, triathletes, and mid-distance runners is similar to over-speed training for sprinters. These training techniques will significantly improve speed.

Running intervals will reduce time per mile in marathons. And over-speed training will reduce time in the shorter sprints. All athletes participating in sports requiring running speed should consider including over-speed training into their fitness plan.

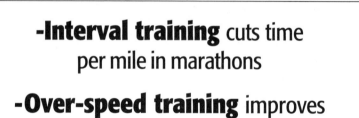

-Interval training cuts time
per mile in marathons

-Over-speed training improves
40 yd dash time

Elite sprinters seeking to cut micro seconds off their time in the 100–meter and 200–meter sprints use over-speed training. Experts claim over-speed training can significantly increase speed.

Over-speed training is based on the theory that the running pace can be improved by training at a faster pace (with some type of speed-assisted device) than you are capable of running. And this works! Even a near 50 year-old masters sprinter like me can improve speed with over-speed training.

For sprinters, over-speed training can be accomplished by running downhill on a surface with a small degree slope. Too much slope can be harmful to the knees. The slope from the center of a football field to the sidelines (drainage slope) is good. Also, a 30 foot piece of surgical tubing can used to pull sprinters for an assisted 10-meter boost. Over-speed training tricks the brain into thinking that you can run faster. I know this works, because I have tried it myself.

Over-speed training devices and speed development resources may be purchased at the following Websites: www.springcoathletics.com, www.ontrackandfield.com, www.gillathletics.com, www.performbetter.com.

Interval Training for Distance Runners

Marathoners. Try this workout to improve your time per mile. Add the following interval/sprint over-speed training program two days a week.

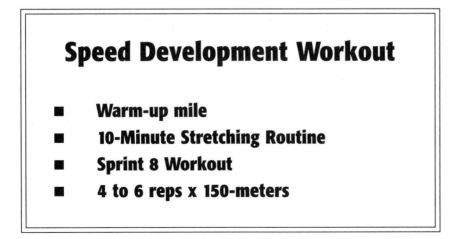

Speed Development Workout

- **Warm-up mile**
- **10-Minute Stretching Routine**
- **Sprint 8 Workout**
- **4 to 6 reps x 150-meters**

Walk-back and fully recover on the Sprint 8 Workout and the 150-meter intervals. Resist the temptation to make this an endurance-building program. Think "speed development and technique" only with this workout.

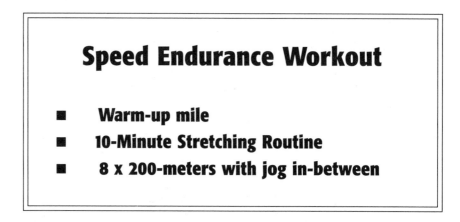

Speed Endurance Workout

- **Warm-up mile**
- **10-Minute Stretching Routine**
- **8 x 200-meters with jog in-between**

Run 200-meters in 28 to 40 seconds, jog at a slow pace the next 200-meters (this completes one lap on a 400-meter track). Sprint the second 200-meters, jog 200-meters. Repeat for four laps total, or eight repetitions of the fast 200s.

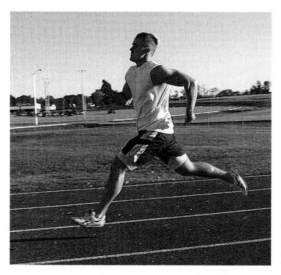

Casey Childers, former college defensive back, uses Synergy Fitness techniques to prepare for professional football.

Secret Weapons in Speed Development

Strong and flexible hip flexors and hamstrings, reducing negative foot speed, and over-speed training are important factors in speed development. Hip flexors are located at the very top and outside of your legs. Hip flexor raises do the job. Sit on the edge of the leg extension machine as shown. Raise the knee high as possible using the top part of your thigh to perform the work.

Hip Flexor Raises

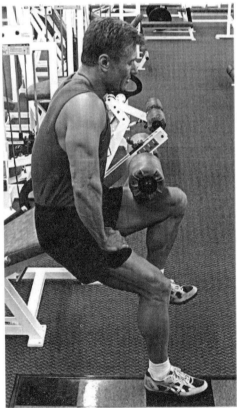

Start

Raised position

Your hamstrings should be 75 to 80 percent as strong as your quadriceps (thighs) in a leg extension to leg curl strength test. Experts report that most athletes have hamstrings that are typically only 50 percent as strong as the quads. Chapter 10, Tactical Weight Training, offers a detailed hamstring development program.

Note: The 10-Minute Stretching Routine needs to have equal emphasis with strength development of the hamstrings.

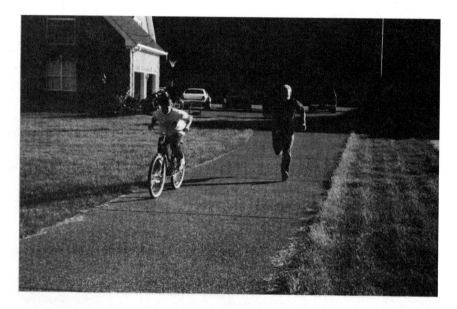

Mickey Miller formed a Synergy Fitness Group with fellow police officers. Mickey is shown sprinting while Darlene Sanders sprints using a bicycle. Both of them are accomplishing the Sprint 8 Workout, which can be done in various ways.

Incorrect—foot down

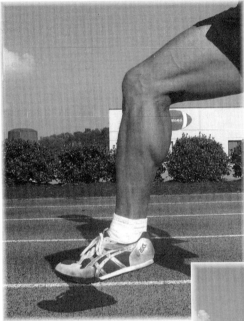

Correct—foot up
"dorsiflexed"

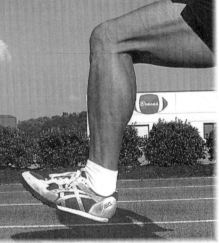

Negative Foot Speed

One of the most common mistakes made by sprinters, mid-distance, and long-distance runners is improper foot position while running. Negative foot speed is created when proper foot and ankle mechanics are not practiced.

Information about
Masters Track and
Field may be
obtained at
www.masterstrack.com,
and www.usatf.org.

The foot should be "dorsiflexed" when running. This means the foot should be turned up (and cocked) and ready to fire when it hits the ground. Running with the foot pointed downward is like throwing a baseball without using the wrist. The prior photos illustrate proper "dorsiflexed" foot positioning for running the Sprint 8 Workout.

Negative foot speed can be eliminated by practicing the rule "foot-up, knee-up, hip-up." Run in the "dorsiflexed" position, with high knee action, and the hips slightly "thrust" forward. The goal is for the foot to strike mid-foot, not on the toes.

Track and Field— The Oldest Sport in History

Track may be the best "second sport" for athletes participating in sports that require running speed. The 2001 Super Bowl champions, the Baltimore Ravens, had more track and field talent than any other team, with eight track stars (*Track & Field News*, 2001).

Since most sports require running speed, quickness and speed endurance, track is an excellent choice as the "second sport" for most athletes.

Masters Track and Field

Runners over age 30, former athletes, and anyone wishing to use healthy competition for inspiration and additional motivation should check out Masters Track and Field. Masters Track and Field is a division of USA Track & Field and has officially sanctioned events.

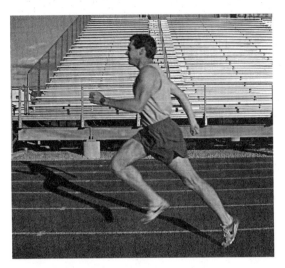

Leon Hoover, age 43, comments on sprinting, "The Sprint 8 Workout amazingly increases my endurance very quickly. All distance runners should try the Sprint 8 Workout for a month, and they will permanently add this to their training."

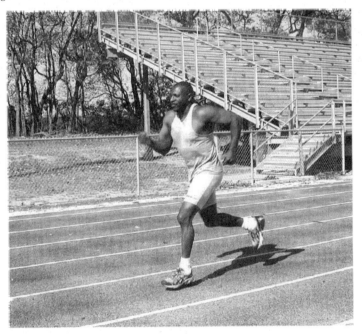

Paul Williams, age 40, comments on the Sprint 8 Workout, "I feel great when I run sprints. It keeps the weight off. And I can eat what I want when I do the Sprint 8 Workout."

Conclusion

Throughout this book, high-intensity anaerobic training has been discussed because anaerobic training is the missing ingredient in most fitness plans. And clearly, it takes anaerobic exercise aimed at the Target Zone—focusing on training fast-twitch muscle fiber IIx—to increase growth hormone naturally. Whether your focus is losing weight, improving fitness, getting ready for the next season, anti-aging, or anti–middle aging, anaerobic exercise is the number one fitness training method to achieve the benefits of Synergy Fitness.

Research is conclusive: anaerobic training significantly increases the release of growth hormone in your body. Anaerobic training is the toughest part of any Strategic Fitness Plan. But it is absolutely essential. Give it a try. It may be slightly painful during the 20 minute workout—but you will love the results!

9

Plyo-Power

Power and strength are not the same—power is strength in action. Power is how strong you are during the game. And fast, explosive power is the goal, and it is delivered by the fast-twitch muscle fiber in your body (Chapter 4).

High school athletes want fast-twitch muscle fiber to make the starting lineup. Olympians want fast muscle fiber to win the gold. And everyone interested in reversing the effects of aging (including middle aging) need fast-twitch muscle fiber to accomplish growth hormone releasing anaerobic exercise.

Plyometric training is the champion at developing fast-twitch IIa muscle fiber, and the super fast IIx muscle fiber.

Researchers demonstrate that regardless of age and physical condition, a total fitness plan should have exercises to improve power and develop fast-twitch muscle fiber.
(Physio-pathologic aspects of aging—possible influence of physical training on physical fitness, 2000, Kostka).

All Ages Benefit from Plyometrics

Children can increase bone density, strength, and power through plyometric jump drills, (*Jumping improves hip and lumbar spine bone mass in prepubescent children: a randomized trial*, 2001, Fuchs).

Adolescent girls that participate in plyometric training increase bone density, (*Effects of plyometric jump training on bone mass in adolescent girls*, 2000, Witzke).

ACL Knee Injury Warning:

Plyometric drills may aid in the prevention of ACL (anterior cruciate ligament) injuries—prevalent in female soccer players. Drills must be performed with adequate warm-up and a gradual build-up period because lateral movements may cause ACL injury.
See www.coachr.org/pep.htm
for an ACL injury-reduction training program designed for female soccer players.

Premenopausal women maintain strength and power with plyometric training. And continued training reduces the risk factor later in life, (*Detraining reverses positive effects of exercise on the musculoskeletal system in premenopausal women*, 2000, Winters).

Senior men and women need power and strength. Researchers report that the elderly are as responsive to strength training as younger adults, (*Applied physiology of strength and power in old age*, 1994, Young). Clearly, strength and power do not need to be forgotten after the competitive days of youth are over.

Plyometrics

Plyometric drills typically involve jumping, skipping, and hopping, but may take many different forms. The activities target fast-twitch IIa and IIx muscle fiber. In creating a plyometric drill, coaches take the important movement specific to a certain sport and create an exercise to develop strength and speed from that one movement.

For example, any sport needing increased speed would break down the common movements and segment them into drills for the various aspects of sport-specific running; cutting in football, stealing base in baseball, running while dribbling in basketball. Various exercises to target all three muscle fiber types of the muscle group used in that sport would be developed.

The basic plyometric drills in this chapter are helpful for sports requiring running speed.

Plyometrics are performed by set/reps similar to weightlifting. There are many different forms of plyometrics. Karate kicks, in many respects, are standing plyometrics. Jumping drills are plyometrics. Plyometrics can be performed almost anywhere.

Most plyometric drills in this chapter are moving forward and typically cover 15-yards followed by a walk-back to the start for the recovery.

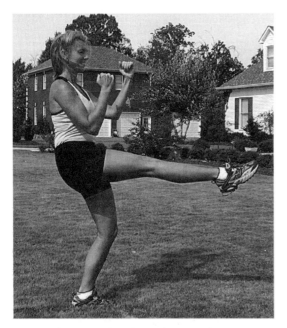

*Personal trainer, Bambi LaFont, performs
karate kicks and plyometric bounding.*

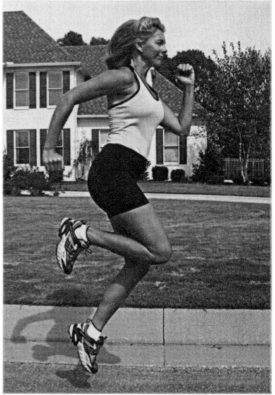

The following chart outlines the Plyo-Power development workout that is programmed into the Strategic Fitness Plans in Chapter 11.

Power Building Plyometrics	
Plyometric Kicks	**Workout:**
Front karate kicks	1 set / 10 kicks -*each leg*
Side karate kicks	1 / 10 kicks
Back kicks	1 / 10 kicks
Plyometric Drills	
High knees	1 to 2 sets/ 15 yards
Butt slaps	1-2 / 15 yds
Wall slides	1-2 / 15 yds
Lunges	1-2 / 15 yds
Optional Plyometrics	
High skips bounding	1 / 15 yds

Beginning with Standing Plyometrics, perform one set of 10 karate kicks—front, side, and back as illustrated in the next three pages. The movements should be fast. However, make sure you have warmed up (by raising your body temperature) before making quick movements. The 90 percent extension rule applies with karate kicks—during the kicks; hold back from a 100 percent extension that can cause injury.

Karate Front Kicks

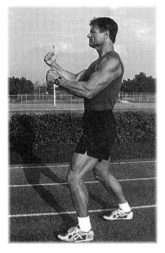
Start

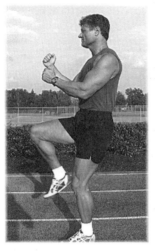
Raise knee

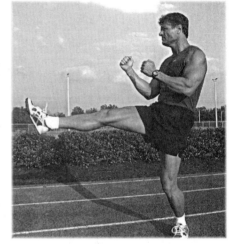
Front kick waist level

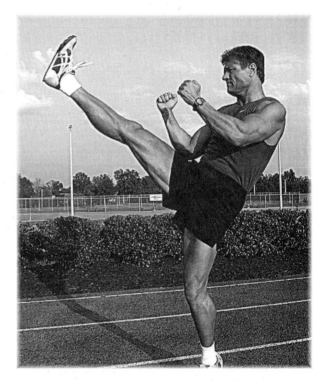
Advanced front kick

Karate Side Kicks

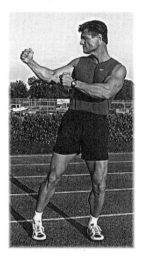 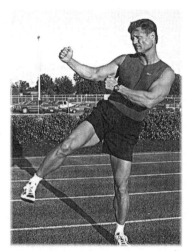 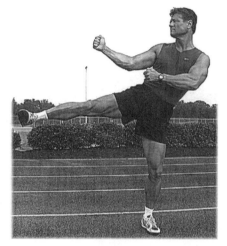

Start   Cock leg   Fire kick to waist level

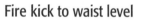

Advanced side kick

Karate Back-Kicks

Start

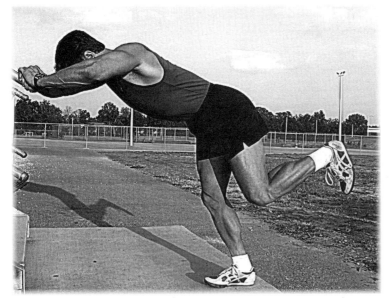

Back kick to waist level

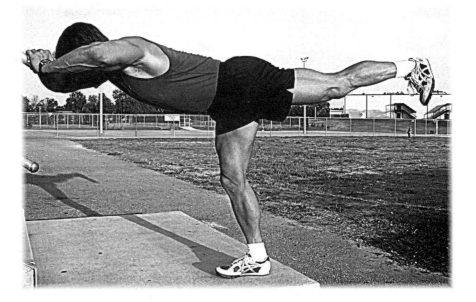

Plyometric Drills

Once plyometric kicks have been accomplished, it is time to perform the plyometric drills.

Initially, perform only one set of plyometric drills covering 10-yards. Progressively build to two sets of 15-yards with a walk-back recovery in-between. This segment should only take 10-minutes initially and build to 20-minutes.

With all plyometric drills, there should be lots of leg action (up and down). However, the progress forward should be equal to the speed of walking.

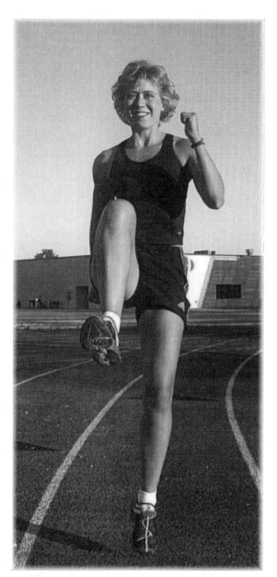

Plyometric High Knees demonstrated by IFPA certified personal trainer, Melanie Joyner.

High Knees

Run forward while raising knees high. Make sure the thigh of the raised knee is at least parallel to the track on each repetition.

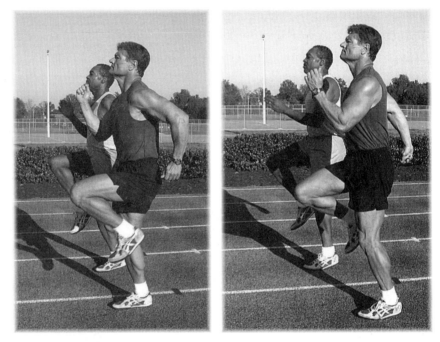

Plyometric High Knees shown with my running partner, Nate Robertson.

Butt Slaps

This drill is typically called butt slaps or butt kickers. Whatever the name, it's a great developer of fast-twitch leg muscles. This drill is especially valuable for the athletes wanting to improve speed. Run forward by raising the back foot as high as possible without raising the knee. Important: keep knees pointed downward during the entire drill.

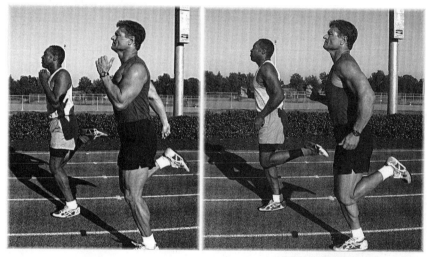

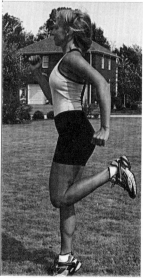

Don't get in a hurry with butt slaps. Move fast to activate the fast-twitch muscle in an up-and-down motion with your feet, but actual progress forward should be equal to the speed of walking.

Plyometrics may be easily performed at home in the yard.

Wall Slides

This drill has been called wall slides, glass wall and fast feet. This drill is halfway between the high knee drill and the butt slaps drill. While moving forward, the knee is brought upward and high, while the foot is limited to coming up in a straight path directly under the body. This drill is called the "wall slide" because you visualize an imaginary wall (from head to toe) directly behind you as you move forward.

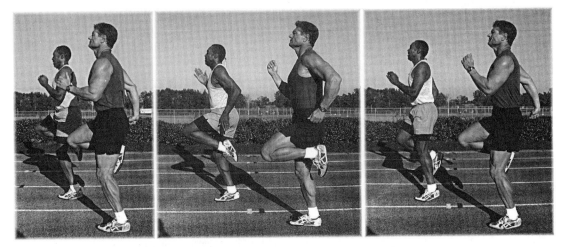

Nate Robertson helps demonstrate wall slides.

Lunges

Lunges are performed by taking steps forward at a slow-walking pace. With hands on hips, take a giant step forward and dip until the forward thigh becomes parallel with the track. Continue walking forward with the reaching lunge steps.

Lunge forward. Dip rear knee as you walk forward.

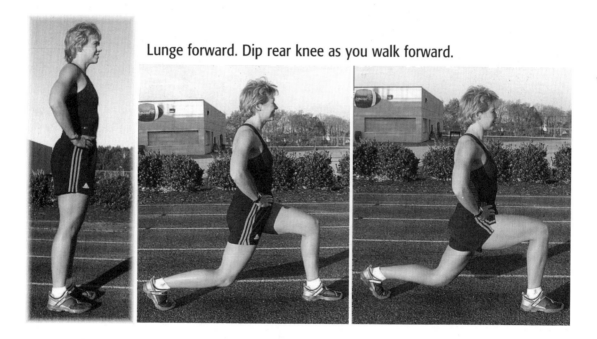

Advanced Plyometrics—Bounding

Bounding has several forms. The Synergy Fitness method is easy. Remember how to skip? Just skip, except at the top of the skip—jump upward as high as possible. Landing can be tough on the ankles, so before you add this plyometric drill to your plan, make sure you have been performing plyometrics for at least 90 days.

High Skips Bounding

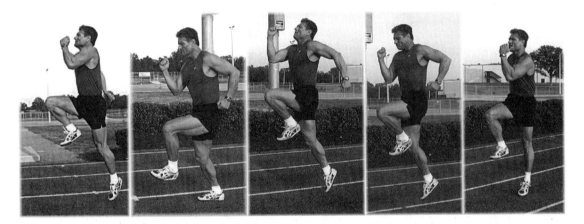

Scheduling Plyometric Drills

Plyometric drills should become a regular part of your Strategic Fitness Plan at least one day per week—beginning with Fitness Level Two. And weight-plyos should be added as the first 3-5 reps per set during resistance training. You can also multi-task plyometric drills with aerobic training, by limiting the walk-back to less than 1-minute.

Developing Power with Plyo-Weight Training

Plyo-weight training is a term used to describe applying explosive plyometric training technique to weightlifting. This method multi-tasks two types of exercise for efficiency by adding plyometric type movements (fast-twitch muscle development) to weightlifting (slow-twitch muscle).

A plyo-lift involves a 2 second pause at the bottom of a lift, followed by a quick 90 percent extension of the weight. The down movement should be similar to the traditional weightlifting tempo of a 3-4 second pace. The pause should be longer than normal (2 seconds). The up movement should be fast and explosive to the 90 percent extension point. The final 10 percent of the extension should be at a normal pace.

Plyo-weight training is for individuals with weight training experience. If you are a newcomer to resistance training, you should wait a few months before adding plyo-weights to your workout.

When performance of traditional weight training, in improving the vertical jump, is compared with "weight-plyos" performance, weight-plyos come out on top. Researchers demonstrated that after completing eight weeks of squat jumps (plyos), versus squats and leg presses, the plyometric squat jumps outperformed classical weightlifting. The difference in performance of the squat jumps was described as "significant" by the researchers, (*Effects of ballistic training on preseason preparation of elite volleyball players*, 1999, Newton). Traditional weight training improves strength, and weight-plyos develop power. Both forms of training need to be included in a comprehensive fitness plan.

Researchers show that plyometrics and weight training compliment each other in a total fitness model. (Weight and plyometric training: effects on eccentric and concern force production, 1996, Wilson).

Plyometric drills in this chapter primarily target leg muscles, although the entire body gets worked during these drills. Plyometric training is also effective for the upper body, (*Stretch-shortening drills for the upper extremities: theory and clinical application,* 1993, Wilk).

The weight-plyos method programmed for your Strategic Fitness Plan may be accomplished several ways. Weight-plyos can be performed on the last weight training set for individual body parts. However, the preferred method is to perform the first 30 percent of the reptitions on every set (usually 3-5 reps) with weigh-plyo techniques. Once the fast-twitch IIa and IIx muscle fibers are exhausted from the weight-plyos early in the set, then revert to the "moderate tempo" to finish the set and exhaust the slow-twitch muscle fiber.

Weight-plyos are a great way to shock your body out of training plateaus caused by muscle memory (Chapter 10). You may even consider incorporating one entire training session in the weight-plyo form for a workout every month or so—especially when experiencing a training plateau.

Since muscle fiber composition is somewhat similar in most people (Chapter 4). Most have approximately 50 percent slow-twitch muscle fiber, 30 percent fast-twitch IIa fiber, and 20 percent super fast IIx fiber. It's reasonable to have a fitness plan that spends 50 percent of training time on slow-twitch muscle development (jogging, long-distance training, traditional weightlifting). Then, 30 percent of training time should be on fast-twitch IIa development (plyo-weights, intervals); and 20 percent of training time on the super fast IIx muscle fiber (quick-burst exercises, sprinting of all sports, martial arts).

Following this formula, 30 percent of your weightlifting should be performed with plyometric techniques. So if you perform the first 30 percent of your reps (first 3 reps on a 10 rep set, first 4 on 12 reps) with weight-plyo techniques, this would accomplish this objective.

Isshinryu 90 Percent Extension Principle

The founder of Isshinryu Karate, Master Tatsuo Shimabuku (1906–1975), designed his form of marital arts to be a lifelong method of training by taking into consideration the injury factor associated with fast, hard, full extension of the legs and arms during kicks and punches. To prevent injury and increase power, the karate master developed a rule that should also be applied to plyo-weight training.

Master Shimabuku declared that all Isshinryu Karate punches and kicks would be limited to 90 percent extension. Applying this same principle with weight-plyos should help avoid injury while achieving the benefits of fast-twitch muscle development.

Bench-Press Plyos

Plyo-weights techniques work well with press and push types of exercises like bench press, leg press, and the various shoulder presses. Using the bench press as an example; lower the bar to your chest, pause 2 seconds, and explode the weight upward quickly and powerfully toward the Isshinryu 90 percent arm extension point.

At this point, let the arms extend naturally the remaining 10 percent to the up position. This method clearly works fast-twitch lla, and perhaps the super fast IIx muscle fiber that frequently goes untouched in most gyms.

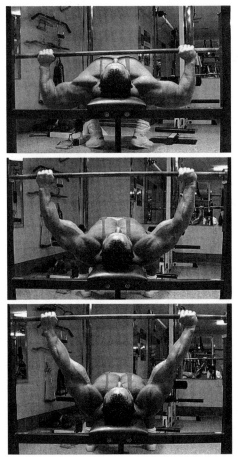

Pause in the lowered position 2 seconds

Explode to 90 percent extension

Complete the full extension before next rep

The preferred Synergy Fitness method is accomplished by using weight-plyos on the first 3-5 reps of every set. This is easily done on press and push types of exercises. Pull types of exercises like pull downs, cable rows, and curls, offer more challenge in working fast-twitch muscle fiber. It can be done, but the pulling movements are not nearly as explosive as the press type of exercises.

I do not think that Louie Simmons calls his weight program "plyo-weight training," but his methods sound similar. Louie is a power lifter who squatted over 900 pounds at age 52. He was stronger at 52 than at 42, and stronger at 42 than at 32. His training plan works very well.

His training program consists of training four times a week—two days of upper body exercise and two days of lower body. He also alternates a heavy day with an "explosive day." Clearly, workouts that include weight-plyos for fast-twitch muscle development yield positive results.

Developing Power with Plyo-Lifts

Increasing power will typically improve athletic performance. And many strength coaches prefer Olympic type lifts for developing power. One of these lifts—the clean, meets the requirement for the physically mature athlete. Power cleans (slightly modified for safety) are programmed for Fitness Level Five—for college and professional athletes in off-season training.

Power Cleans

Power cleans are slightly different from the Olympic version of cleans, which begin at the floor and move up to the finish position in one movement. Power cleans have been modified over the years for safety. The modified version begins at the waist. Note: Many NFL team strength coaches have their athletes begin just below the knees for the extra thrust of the movement.

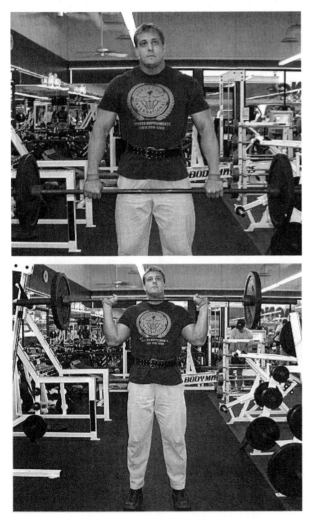

Extra caution needs to be taken with this lift, even for well trained athletes. The initial movement from the floor to the start position needs to be performed with a straight back as shown (right) to avoid injury.

Power cleans and Olympic lifts are good for building power. However, there are problems with these lifts. The main issue is that many younger athletes have been injured performing Olympic lifts because they do not yet have the muscular structure to support this type of lifting.

Jason McCarver demonstrates power cleans.

Personally, I cannot manage the weight necessary for these strenuous lifts. However, the weight-plyos method works well for me. The Strategic Fitness Plan—Level Five (for college and professional athletes) includes Olympic type lifts one day a week. For the other four levels, weight-plyos achieve the Target Zone Method of building fast-twitch muscles.

Back straight   **Start**   **Out and up thrust**

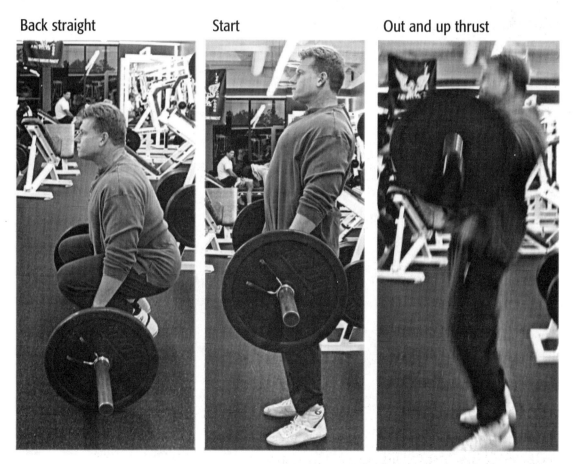

Dr. Don Buchanan demonstrates power cleans.

Push Presses

Push presses resemble the Olympic clean and jerk lift. Hammer Strength makes a machine for push presses called the Hammer Jammer. This is an excellent piece of equipment for sports training.

The first movement is to bend the knees as shown and explode the dumbbells (or barbell) upward.

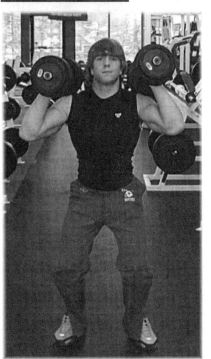

Start

Lower the body and explode the weight to 90 percent extension.

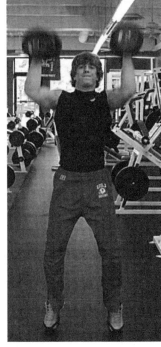

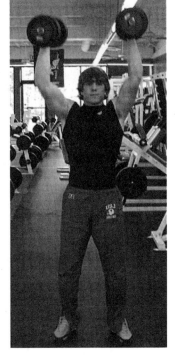

Randy Sheffield, All-Regional Defensive Player and Honorable Mention All-State football player demonstrates push presses.

Clean and Jerk

The Clean and Jerk is an Olympic lift consisting of two parts. The Clean, which gets the weight to the shoulders, followed by the Jerk. The Jerk is performed by quickly pressing the weight overhead while splitting the legs. This advanced lift can be dangerous if not performed correctly. Only Level Five athletes should perform this lift.

Kirk Pafford demonstrates the Clean and Jerk.

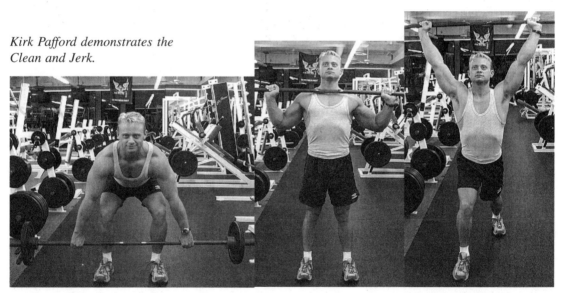

Start   First lift (Clean)   Finish lift (Jerk)

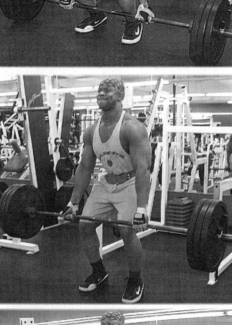

Dead Lift

The dead lift is a demanding advanced exercise requiring a support belt for safety. Use the reverse grip on one hand and keep the back straight as the pull upward is made. Terrance Copeland demonstrates the correct form for a power dead lift.

Initial pull forward keeping
the back straight

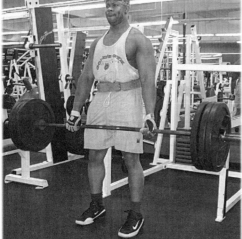

Keep lower back straight

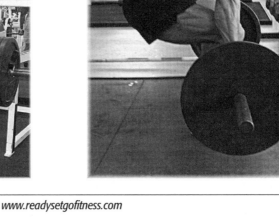

Fitness Routine Training

Fitness routines used in women's fitness competitions target strength, power, flexibility, endurance, and anaerobic development. There should be more encouragement for women and men to participate in this type of comprehensive training and competition.

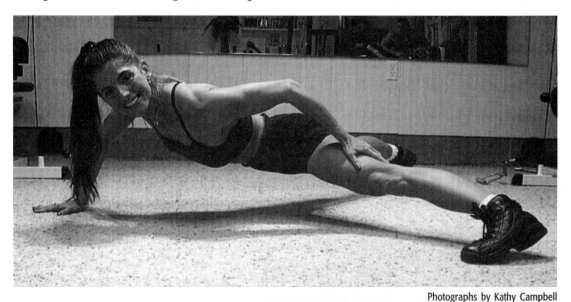

Photographs by Kathy Campbell

Kate Shelby, State Fitness Champion, practices movements for a fitness routine.

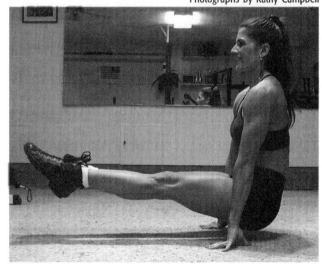

Researchers cite the exercise intensity difference between the 60 to 75 percent range and the 80 percent range as "significant" in obtaining desired results from training. *(The effects of physical training of functional capacity in adults ages 46 to 90: A meta-analysis,* 2000, Lemura).

Conclusion

Researchers show that intensity levels above 80 percent accomplish significantly more than lesser intensities. Plyometrics deliver!

The following chapter, *Tactical Weight Training*, discusses strength training. Then in Chapter 11, the major components of Synergy Fitness will come together to form your Strategic Fitness Plan.

10

Tactical Weight Training

Resistance training with weights or other equipment is essential in achieving the goals of Synergy Fitness. Adding lean muscle through strength training will increase "resting metabolism," and this creates additional synergy in your body to further reduce body fat, (*Grandad, it ain't what you eat, it depends when you eat it—that's how muscles grow!*, 2001, Rennie).

Whether weightlifting in a gym, bowflexing at home, using a universal gym machine in the neighbor's garage, or implementing your Strategic Fitness Plan with free weights at home, resistance training has wonderful synergy benefits.

Adding New Muscle Makes Your Body a Fat Eating Machine

The most efficient way to permanently lose excess body fat, according to researchers, is to implement a "diet with exercise" strategy. The idea of losing body fat without a strategy of developing muscle is not effective.

Researchers show that maintaining and adding muscle through strength training synergistically increases "metabolic rate, and this enhances your body's ability to reduce fat during rest," (*Physical activity, overweight, and obesity*, 2000, Stromme). Resistance training is a major component of the Synergy Fitness.

Regardless of age and physical condition, medical research shows that a comprehensive fitness plan should include resistance training for strength and muscle development. You can join the most expensive gym in your area or purchase some free weights at a yard sale, but resistance training needs to be in your fitness plan.

Resistance Training Principles

Some methods of weight training will reach GH-release benchmarks. Some will not. Weightlifting and other forms of resistance training following the prescribed methods in this chapter will help you reach GH-release benchmarks—muscle-burn (lactic acid), oxygen debt (out-of-breath at the end of an exercise), adrenal release (slightly painful), and increased body temperature (sweating).

It's simple—increasing growth hormone means more muscle tone and development, and less fat.

PRINCIPLES FOR SUCCESSFUL RESISTANCE TRAINING

1. Isolation - of the muscle group being exercised.

2. Exhaustion - of the muscles being worked during every set.

3. Aerobic tempo - between sets. Only rest briefly between sets. (1-minute is ideal, 2-minutes maximum)

Isolation

Isolating a muscle group during weightlifting makes a huge difference in results because it makes you zone in and target the specific muscle being worked. The goal is simply to isolate only one target muscle group that you are training. The hard part is to position the exercise to minimize any other muscle groups from assisting the targeted muscle.

Other muscle groups try to assist as the targeted muscle becomes fatigued, especially at the end of a set. If you let other muscles assist, the impact of training is decreased. This is the most difficult aspect of weight training technique. Focus on not allowing other muscles to assist when the targeted muscle becomes fatigued.

For example, countless times, I have talked with individuals, even serious bodybuilders and professional athletes, who cannot seem to build biceps. This is an easy fix! Invariably, bicep curls were being performed with the wrists bent toward the body rather than straight. This positions the forearms to do much of the work, rather than the biceps.

ISOLATION PRINCIPLE dictates slightly bending the wrist backwards during curls (away from the body). This prevents the forearms from assisting, thereby isolating the biceps to do the work (and receive the full benefit of the exercise). The following photos show the correct and incorrect positions to isolate biceps.

Incorrect—wrist bent. Bicep not isolated, forearm doing the work.

Correct—wrist slightly bent. Isolation is on the bicep, not the forearm.

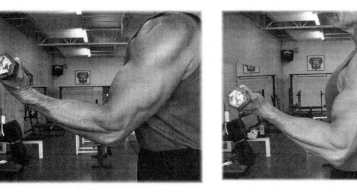

"SLOW MOVEMENT" WEIGHT TRAINING?

Slow movement weight training is a new trend in some gyms. The idea is to very slowly lift weights. This method will assist in isolating the muscle group being worked. However, there is no scientific magic behind "slow movement" lifting. If you are correctly isolating muscle groups during training (and keeping muscle groups isolated during the set), then a moderate tempo works well to target slow-twitch muscle fiber.

Exhaustion

Exhaustion of the muscle group during every set must occur—or don't count the set (and repeat the set). This is a good rule to follow and will yield great results.

If you have not experienced "going to exhaustion" during every set, you will be amazed at the results. Typically, individuals limit the exercise to a prescribed number of repetitions (reps) when more could be done.

Researchers show that multiple sets per body part produce greater strength gains than one set per body part. (Borst, 2001).

EXHAUSTION PRINCIPLE dictates squeezing out 11 or 12 reps, or more if possible. If you can perform 13 to 15 reps, it is time to increase resistance (add 5-10 lbs) during the next set, and the next workout.

Aerobic Tempo:
1-Minute Rest Between Sets is Ideal

Make weight training an aerobic workout. You can multi-task aerobic exercise and resistance training simultaneously by only resting briefly between sets. Ideal rest between sets is 30 seconds to 1-minute, and 2-minutes should be the maximum. Multi-tasking strength training with cardio not only saves time, it produces great results. This method of multi-tasking training methods also increases the potential for achieving GH-release benchmarks.

Not effective is the style of weight training where an individual performs a set, stops at 10 reps (when fifteen could have been done) and rests several minutes between sets. This will not increase GH release or burn many calories. It is okay to rest more than 1-minute between training body parts during split training routines. However, while working a body part—stay focused on the 1-minute rest between sets.

On days when I feel like I need more than a minute's rest between sets, I silently recite a personal mental trigger to "get tough, get focused, and get going" with intensity. I take a deep breath and say to myself, "Ready, Set, GO!" and then I start the set.

Target Zone of Resistance Training

Resistance training has two Target Zones in every muscle group being worked. Resistance training should target slow-twitch, type I muscle fiber for strength improvement. And the first 3-5 reps per set performed with weight-plyo technique targets the fast-twitch fiber. This method will work most of your muscle fiber rather than only the slow-twitch fiber worked by traditional resistance training.

Fatiguing muscles, raising body temperature and achieving muscle burn are the goals during every set. Working hard enough to create the need to catch your breath during the set will achieve GH-release benchmarks.

The Target Zone Training Method is discussed in detail in Chapter 4.

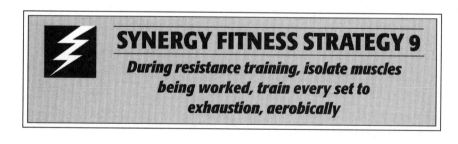

SYNERGY FITNESS STRATEGY 9

During resistance training, isolate muscles being worked, train every set to exhaustion, aerobically

The Ultimate Weightlifting Question: What's Best– High Reps/Low Weight, or Low Reps /Heavy Weight?

The answer to this question is . . . yes! Research shows that both methods are effective. The underlying principle is in the "intensity of the exercise" not a precise number of repetitions. Researchers show that eight reps (at 80 percent of one rep maximal lift) versus 16 reps (at 40 percent of max) obtain equal results in women during six months of training, (*Musculoskeletal responses to high- and low-intensity resistance training in early postmenopausal women*, 2000, Bemben).

Following the principles of Exhaustion, Isolation, and Aerobic Tempo, weight training will achieve the intensity necessary for optimum results.

Breathing During Resistance Training

The rule on breathing during resistance training is simple. Exhale when the repetition is the most difficult. Inhale on the return movement. Example: On press type exercises such as the bench press or shoulder press, exhale on the press up movement and inhale while lowering the weight. On pull downs or cable rows, exhale on the pull in movement and inhale as you release the weight.

Fitness Center Membership?

Strength training can be performed with resistance in many forms besides weightlifting in a fitness center. Time-crunched adults may not have the time to drive to a gym. If you are self-disciplined, you *can* make a strategic fitness plan work at home.

Dr. Keith Williams, a physician with a full-time Ob-Gyn practice, the chairperson of deacons at his church, and an active parent of four children, makes four hours a week for the Strategic Fitness Plan Level Two. He uses Wal-Mart free weights, a bench, and has 70-yards marked in his front yard for his Sprint 8 Workouts.

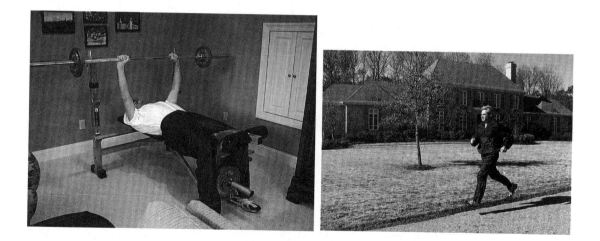

However, a fitness center membership will provide a certain amount of peer pressure that can be positive. Research shows that there is an important social aspect associated with a fitness center membership (once you get to know some friends there), and these relationships are sometimes effective in maintaining consistency.

How you are motivated may be a necessary question to ask yourself concerning a fitness center membership. Making fitness training convenient is an important factor in maintaining a long-term program.

If you enjoy social relationships and need pressure for motivation, consider a gym membership, walking club, running club, or you could start your own Synergy Fitness Group and recruit some friends or colleagues to begin with you. If you respond to competition, place yourself in a competitive environment—check out Masters Track and Field on the Internet (www.usatf.org or www.masterstrack.com) or other masters' event competitions.

If you need peer pressure *and* competition for motivation, as I do, then consider a gym membership. However, if the fitness center membership is simply not in your budget, you can easily make the fitness plan work with an inexpensive set of weights from Wal-Mart, or find them at a yard sale. You can do it!

Repetition Tempo

With the exception of explosive weight-plyos, the basic tempo for weightlifting repetitions should be approximately 2 seconds going up, and 3-4 seconds going down for press-type movements (bench press, shoulder press, leg press).

On pull-type exercises, you pull in for 2-3 seconds, and the release out should last 3-4 seconds (pull downs, cable pulls, curls).

Whole or Split Body Routines?

"Whole-body" resistance training is prescribed for Fitness Levels One and Two. "Split-body" routines begin at Level Three because the workload of Level Three is too great to be performed by all body parts during a single day.

During the first five months of weight training, research shows (for young healthy women), that whole-body routines slightly outperform split-body routines, (*Comparison of whole and split weight training routines in young women, 1994, Calder*). Whole body routines are preferred for newcomers to resistance training.

WHOLE VS. SPLIT ROUTINE COMPARISONS
20 weeks of weight training for newcomers

Results:	Whole-body	Split-body
Leg muscle increase	4.9 %	1.7 %
Overall muscle increase	4.1	2.6
Decrease in fat	1.1 (loss)	1.3 (loss)

Middle-aged and older men participating in strength training research, experience "significant" gains in strength and power in 16 weeks of training. (Effects of strength training on muscle power and serum hormones in middle-aged and older men, 2000, Izquierdo).

Weight Training is Anti-Aging

Weight training is beneficial for women with chronic heart failure (CHF), according to recent medical research. In 2001, researchers studied the impact of strength training on 16 older women with chronic heart failure.

The results? Exercise was "well-tolerated" and improved strength by 8.8 percent, endurance improved by 66 percent, and type I muscle fiber increased 16 percent during the 10 week study period, (*Randomized controlled trial of progressive resistance training to counteract the skeletal muscle myopathy of chronic heart failure*, 2001, Pu).

In another study, 40 adults with an average age of 69, were divided into two groups and completed either six months of resistance training or six months of endurance training. Researchers determined that the endurance-trained group improved "oxidative capacity" (the body's ability to supply oxygen to the blood) by 31 percent, but the resistance-trained group improved 57 percent. The weight-training group also experienced a 10 percent increase in muscle size, (*Large energetic adaptations of elderly muscle to resistance and endurance training*, 2001, Jubrias).

The results of these studies are important, if not profound. First, strength training was successful in producing positive results. The endurance group made remarkable improvement, and the resistance-training group almost doubled those results.

Do not drop aerobic training for weight training. Aerobic training is productive. However, you need to consider adding weight training on different days to vary your program and achieve the strength development aspect of Synergy Fitness.

Strength training performed by the elderly produces wonderful results. It increases endurance, normalizes blood pressure, reduces insulin resistance, reduces body fat, increases resting metabolic rate, reduces the risk of falls, and reduces pain in knee joints, (*Strength training in elderly effects on risk factors for age related diseases,* 2000, Hurley).

Weight Training for Children?

Weight training for children has been long debated. Current research provides answers. Researchers at LSU Medical School show that even obese children (ages 7 to 12) benefit from resistance training. After one year of resistance training, children in the study "significantly" reduced fat. And resistance training produced a positive exercise retention factor for the children, (*Safety, feasibility, and efficacy of a resistance training program in preadolescent obese children,* 2000, Sothern).

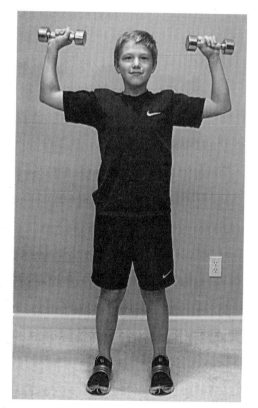

What do pediatricians say about children weightlifting? The American Academy of Pediatrics issued a new position on this subject in June 2001. The report cites the many benefits of strength training for teenagers and even preadolescents. Earlier concerns of injuries to the wrist and back were reported as "largely preventable by avoiding improper lifting techniques, maximal lifts, and improperly supervised lifts."

John Campbell demonstrates shoulder presses.

Does weightlifting stunt growth in children? No, according to the AAP. "Strength training programs do not seem to adversely affect linear growth," (AAP citing "*The effects of a twice-a-week strength training program on children,*" Faigenbaum, 1993).

Will resistance training impact youth sports performance? Yes, in positive ways. The *National Alliance for Youth Sports* recommends strength conditioning by using exercises that require children to control their own body weight rather than using weight training equipment.

There are many ways to use resistance for sport-specific strength development. The *National Alliance for Youth Sports* (www.nays.org) is an excellent organization dedicated to stopping violence in youth sports and **stopping the use of exercise as punishment**. Parents and coaches attending the two-hour NAYS training certification, prior to coaching children, receive basic instruction in using positive teaching fundamentals while coaching.

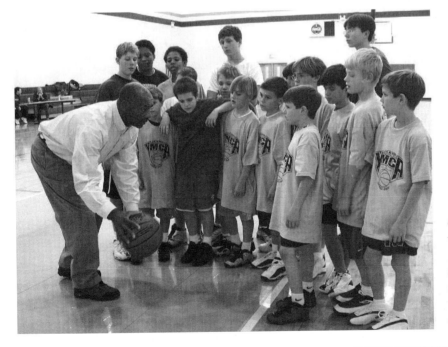

Coach Larry Jones, volunteer coach for over 25 years, uses positive teaching techniques while coaching children.

HIGHLIGHTS OF THE AMERICAN ACADEMY OF PEDIATRICS

Strength Training Recommendations for Children

- Strength training can be safe and effective if proper training techniques and safety guide lines are followed. (Details at AAP Website www.aap.org)
- Exercises should be learned initially without load until technique is learned
- Warm-up and cool-down
- No maximal / single lifts. Perform 8 – 15 repetitions "in good form" during sets
- Avoid competitive lifting, power lifting, body building until reaching physical and skeletal maturity
- Workouts should be 20–30 minutes long targeted at major muscle groups, two to three times a week.

The basic push-up is an example of using the body weight for sports-specific exercise resistance. Some children may be unable to use their body weight in this fashion. And the child may actually need to use weight training at home with lighter weight (perhaps much less than body weight) and high repetitions to build to the point where body weight resistance is achievable for sports participation.

Christine Campbell demonstrates the push-up.

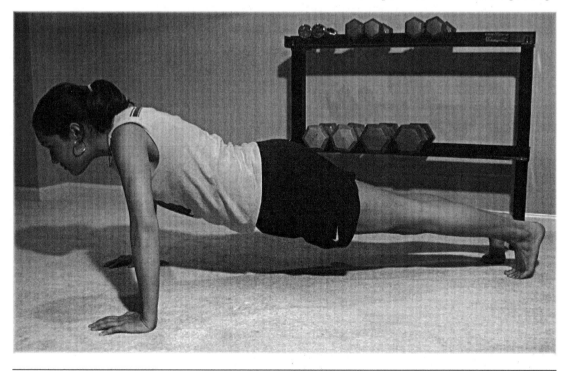

Personal Trainer. Do You Need One?

Personal trainers—if they are qualified, experienced (with your age group), motivated and motivating—can make positive things happen like help jump-start a fitness plan, or assist you through a training plateau. Even the most motivated fitness leaders experience training plateaus from time to time.

How to select a personal trainer? Ask friends at a fitness center who have used a personal trainer. And don't make the decision on the first name you hear. Spend some time with this decision. Make it a deliberate, well thought out decision. Once you have someone in mind, talk to a couple of clients and ask about training philosophy, age group experience, time commitments, certification, and the amount of attention given during training. Be sure that the trainer uses a comprehensive Synergy Fitness type approach.

SOURCES FOR CERTIFIED PERSONAL TRAINERS

ACE American Council on Exercise
45,000 active ACE-Certified Fitness Professionals worldwide
<u>www.acefitness.org</u> San Diego, CA   (800) 825-3636
(Excellent Website)

AFAA Aerobics and Fitness Association of America
150,000 fitness professional worldwide
<u>www.afaa.com</u> Sherman Oaks, CA   (877) 968-7263

IFPA International Fitness Professionals Association
<u>www.ifpa-fitness.com</u> Tampa, Florida (800) 785-1924
(Easy-to-use Website)

Resistance Training Supplements: Which Supplements Really Work?

Advertisements for supplements that promote muscle growth and fat loss to be used with resistance training seem to be everywhere. Many supplements are effective in promoting muscle growth and their benefits are proven by scientific research. And remember, adding muscle makes your body act like a fat eating machine by improving resting metabolism.

SHOULD SUPPLEMENTS BE TAKEN BEFORE OR AFTER TRAINING? A study at the University of Tennessee shows that protein supplements before *and* after training are helpful in promoting growth-oriented hormones during exercise and recovery, (*Dietary supplements and promotion of muscle growth with resistance exercise*, 1999, Kreider).

Significant findings from this study:
- Chromium and vanadyl do not affect muscle growth, as once thought.
- Glutamine, creatine, and calcium beta-HMB have positive outcomes.

PROTEIN SUPPLEMENTS before and after, but especially after training promotes muscle toning and growth. Just remember the GH-release strategies from Chapter 3 no high fat meals one hour before workouts, no sugar for two hours after training, and 25 grams of protein after training.

Be careful to read more than the headlines about protein and other supplements. Recently, headlines read, "Medical Group Warns Against High-Protein Diets." This almost sounds like physicians are against protein in your diet. Actually, the article was concerning research by the

American Heart Association that shows that high-protein diets consisting of protein and lots of fat caused health problems because of the excess fat, not the high protein.

HMB (beta-hydroxy-beta-methylbutyrate) has been shown by researchers to increase lean body mass in several recent studies, (*Over-the-counter supplements and strength training*, 2000, Joyner).

CREATINE promotes growth during resistance training. Many studies show that creatine has the ability to promote muscle growth, whereas androstenedione and pyruvate do not, (*Effects of in-season [5-weeks] creatine and pyruvate supplements on anaerobic performance and body composition in American football players,* 1999, Stone). Creatine increases strength and energy during training. And the additional exercise intensity is what produces the gains.

There are several studies documenting positive affects of protein supplementation after training. (Nutritional supplementation and resistance training exercise: what is the evidence for enhanced skeletal muscle hypertrophy, 2000, Gibala).

Personally, I have negative reactions with creatine supplements. Studies have generally involved young athletes, and I am nearly 50. Perhaps it's the middle age issue causing problems or lack of fluids during training, but creatine makes me gain water weight. And while sprinting (even with extra fluid), I have slightly pulled a hamstring on two different occasions experimenting with creatine supplements. There are reports from a small number of athletes that have experienced muscle cramps and muscle pulls while supplementing with creatine, but recent research contradicts these reports—at least for young athletes.

Research on creatine is still taking place and new studies are produced often. The findings are mixed concerning impact on certain sports. Example: A lead researcher (Mujika) discovered that creatine supplements would not help sprint swimmers, while the sprint performance of "repeated sprints" by soccer players was improved with creatine.

Based on this research, creatine supplements will not help on a 1-rep bench press maximal lift. But creatine may help you raise your training intensity (with repeated bench press sets) and the increase in intensity will build strength.

ANDROSTENE (dione) and (diol) were studied at length in 2000 at East Tennessee State University in the Andro Project. Androstene—made famous by baseball great Mark McGuire—caused a 16 percent testosterone increase after one month of treatment. However, at the end of twelve weeks, testosterone levels dropped to pretreatment levels. Why? The body's own production dropped to compensate for the initial artificial boost from the supplements.

Estrogen-related compounds (negative to muscle growth) increased along with other unfavorable cholesterol increases that raised coronary heart disease risk. Neither strength nor body composition changed during the twelve-week experiment, (*The Andro Project: physiological and hormonal influences of androstenedione supplementation in men 35 to 65 years old participating in a high-intensity resistance training program,* 2000, Broeder).

DHEA produced similar results to the Andro Project. During an eight-week study, DHEA did not increase testosterone, which is positive for muscle growth and the desired outcome of DHEA supplementation, (*Effect of oral DHEA on serum testosterone and adaptations to resistance training in young men,* 1999, Brown).

One group in the study took 50 milligrams of DHEA and it increased androstenedione within 60 minutes, however, it did not increase testosterone.

Another group took 150 milligrams daily along with resistance training. The control group trained as the other group, but only took placebos. The results for the strength training groups (with and without DHEA) were the same. The researchers could only conclude that DHEA does not achieve the desired increase in testosterone.

New Research on Supplements

The GNC web site has information on supplements and drug interactions www.gnc.com. Detailed supplement information is available on an award-winning Website produced by the U.S. Department of Agriculture www.nal.usda.gov/fnic/.

The National Institutes of Health has an Office of Dietary Supplements that is responsible for supporting supplement research and distributing research results. www.dietary-supplements.info.nih.gov.

For specific supplement, health, and fitness questions, the "Go Ask Alice" Web site produced by Columbia University www.goaskalice.columbia.edu/Cat3.html is an excellent source of information. This site provides a question and answer format to address specific issues, including questions typically confidential in nature.

Stretching During Resistance Training

Stretching during resistance training is an absolute must if you want the full benefits of Synergy Fitness. The 10-Minute Stretching Routine targets the lower body and you can achieve synergy by stretching the upper body during resistance training. For example; while working chest, take 30 seconds between one of the sets (during recovery) and perform the javelin chest stretch. The upper body stretching positions are demonstrated in Chapter 6.

Stretch the body part being worked is the rule for stretching the upper body during resistance training. Slowly move into the fully stretched position. Once fully stretched, you will feel the limit and the slight discomfort. Hold for 30 seconds, and slowly ease out of the position. There should be no bouncing in order to reduce risk of injury.

In recent years bodybuilders have begun to add stretching to their weight training. The credit for this productive innovation goes to John Parrillo of Cincinnati, Ohio. He recognized an opportunity that was being missed by many bodybuilders to improve muscle development, definition, and symmetry through flexibility training. And he designed fitness center equipment especially for improving flexibility. Details are available at www.parrillo.com.

Tactical Weight Training

The purpose of this section is to illustrate various resistance-training exercises that target main body parts–chest, back, shoulder, biceps, triceps, quads, hamstrings, calves, abs, and obliques. Specific exercises targeting these key muscle groups are placed in your Strategic Fitness Plan.

Individual body parts serve as the overall Target Zone for these exercises, but remember that you should also **zone-in** on the slow-twitch, fast-twitch IIa, and the super fast-twitch IIx muscle fiber within each muscle group. This will work all of your muscles, ligaments, and joints–and help you get the most benefit from your training time.

Core Exercises

Core exercises are the proven exercises that generally work a major muscle group with one exercise. These are the gold standard of resistance training exercises.

Core exercises will remain in weight-training workouts through the initial eight week training period and beyond. Core exercises, such as bench press, shoulder press, and curls, will be a permanent fixture for all five training levels.

As you progress in Synergy Fitness and become stronger and better conditioned, you will need to add more resistance, (more weight, sets and reps), and additional exercises to continue your progress. The additional exercises are called "finishing exercises."

With each muscle group, there are typically several exercise options to select within the Finishing Exercise group. Finishing exercises are discussed on the following page.

Finishing Exercises

Finishing exercises are used to finish off a body part after the core exercises have been performed. Finishing exercises typically target a specific area within a major body part. Decline press for example, specifically targets the lower chest.

Finishing exercises are in addition to, and always follow core exercises. Here you have options. Finishing exercises may be substituted with other finishing exercises. And the selection based on your preference, as long as the substitution is made within the body part listing.

Some finishing exercises fit better with others because they work the same area. And exercise substitutions are sometimes suggested in the *Body Part Exercise Key*. Example; decline press and dips both work the lower chest so it is suggested that you alternate these two exercises and not do them during the same workout.

Many experienced personal trainers change exercise routines for their clients at different periods to increase muscle stimulation. Muscle memory is a reality, and it can cause some exercises to lose their impact after months of repetition, unless they are changed periodically.

Some finishing exercises require special equipment, however, alternatives are provided for a complete workout—even at home with minimal equipment.

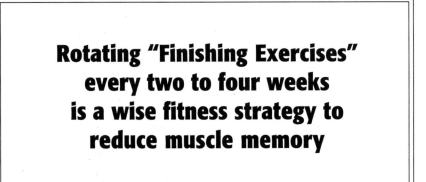

**Rotating "Finishing Exercises"
every two to four weeks
is a wise fitness strategy to
reduce muscle memory**

Body Part Exercise Key

A *Body Part Exercise Key* is provided for training Target Zones (major body parts). The *Keys* list Core Exercises and Finishing Exercises.

To emphasize the strategy that you are to focus on, zone-in, target and really work a specific area of your body, a Synergy Fitness Lightning Bolt is placed on the *Body Part Exercise Keys*. This graphic also divides the core exercises from the finishing exercises. Following the Body Part Exercise Key are the photo-illustrations and descriptions of all the exercises.

Remember, do not simply go through the motion of an exercise. Think Target Zone Training; zone-in on one body part and target all three muscle fibers–slow-twitch, fast-twitch IIa, and super fast IIx muscle fiber within every muscle group. And work the body part with exercises using the three principles: Isolation, Exhaustion, and Aerobic Tempo.

Body part Exercise Key

Targeting Chest

Core
Bench press
Incline press

Finishing
Machine chest flys
Incline dumbbell flys
Decline press or Dips
Cable flys or Cable crossovers
Pullovers or Serratus cable pulls

Bench Press

Bench press is the weight lifting version of the push-up and excellent for **overall chest** development. There are many ways to perform this basic exercise that targets the chest muscles. The bench press is performed with a straight bar on a flat bench (with bar rack) as shown by IFPA certified personal trainer, Melanie Joyner.

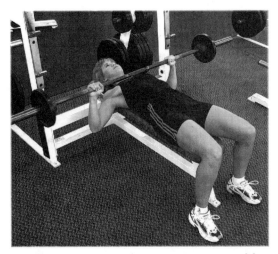
Lower position

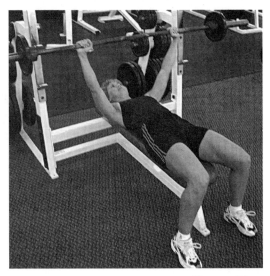
Up position

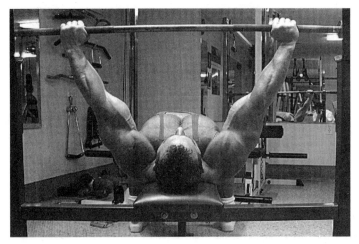

Nick Shelby, nationally ranked bodybuilder, demonstrates the technique of fully extending the arms between repetitions.

Bench Press Alternatives

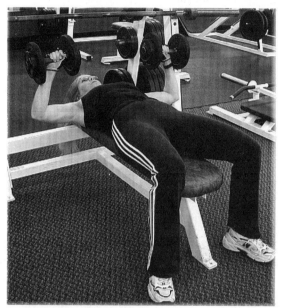

Personal trainer Melissa Marvin,
AFAA certified.

Flat bench dumbbell press
Same as bench press with dumbbells

Machine chest press
on an upright machine

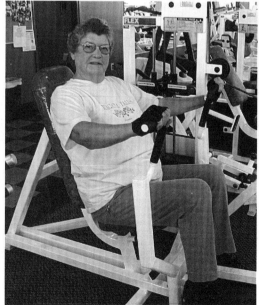

Pat Hutchison

Push-Ups. Great on the Road

The good old push-up is essentially a bench press with body weight resistance to work **overall chest**. Push-ups are limited by having only one level of resistance—body weight. Free weights and resistance machines allow the selection of the right amount of resistance maximizing the results.

In a pinch while traveling, push-ups provide a good chest workout. Next time you are traveling, try the Hotel Room Push-up Routine. Do one push-up, stand, and tap a door facing once. Then do two push-ups, stand, and tap twice. Next, do three and repeat all the way to 10 (total 55 push-ups). I learned this workout from former professional football player, Dale Brady, 30 years ago.

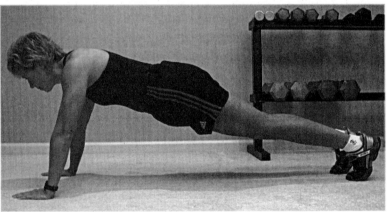

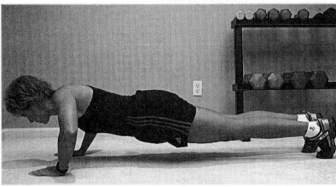

Incline Press

Incline press with a barbell is essentially a bench press on an incline bench. The incline shifts the focus of the exercise to target the **upper chest**. While more difficult than the bench press, this is my personal favorite for chest development.

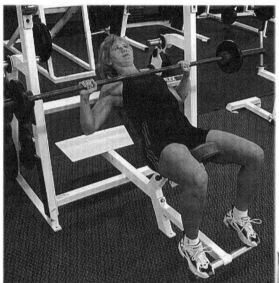

Lower to touch chest

Press up

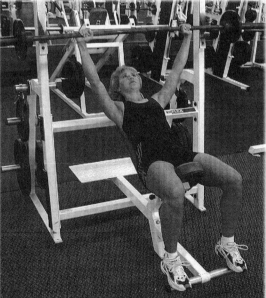

Incline Dumbbell Press

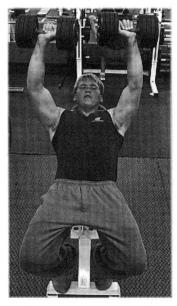 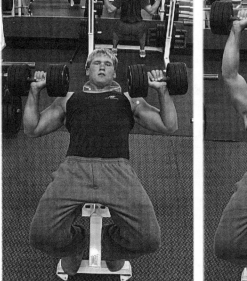 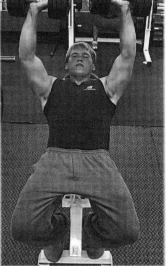

Start   Lower to chest   Up

Incline dumbbell press is demonstrated by Nick Friend. Nick uses the Sprint 8 Workout to promote muscle development and "cutting" for bodybuilding.

Incline Cable Press

Incline cable press targets the **upper chest**. Cable exercises offer benefits to resistance training by adding variety and working muscles at different angles. Cables, like dumbbells, require your muscles to work to stabilize the resistance (in every direction) in addition to the traditional pushing/pulling of weight-lifting. There are great home gym units available that offer cable resistance. And most fitness centers have cable machines. If a gym is not convenient, the Bow-flex unit is excellent for a home (www.bowflex.com) workout.

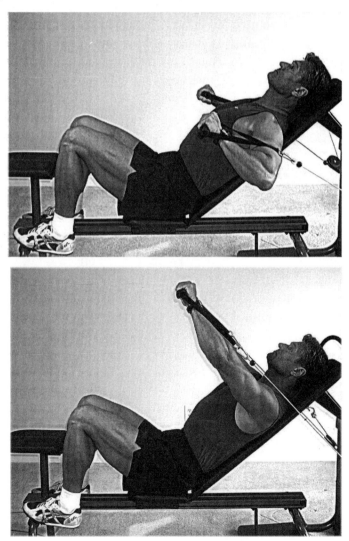

Press up position

Cable Chest Flys

Like all chest flys, cable flys target a specific area of the chest and serve well as a finishing exercise. What is the target area for flys? The rule: if the cable movement is below the chest (as shown below) the **lower chest** receives the focus—If the movement is above the shoulders, the upper chest is the target.

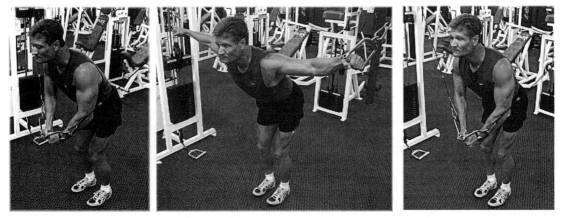

Start   Fly "out" position   Fly "in" position

Cable Crossovers

Cable crossovers are similar to cable chest flys except the arms are bent more at the "out" position and the cables are crossed at the end of every repetition. Palms are faced toward your body during this exercise. And this angle places the resistance on the lower chest.

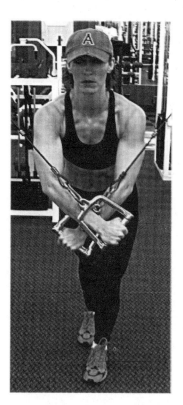

Shay Ingram.

Joan Vidrine demonstrates machine flys.

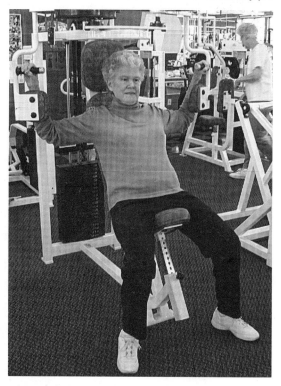

Machine Flys

Machine flys provide a great workout. This angle targets the **lower chest**.

Decline Press

Decline press targets the **lower chest**. This exercise is the same as bench press but on a decline bench.

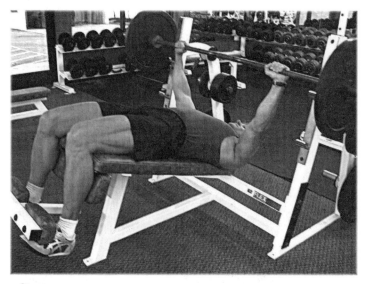

Start

Lower to touch chest

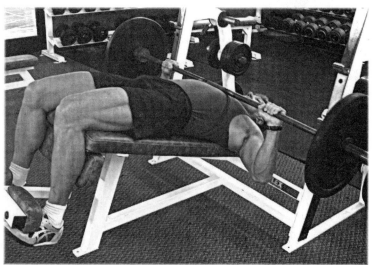

Dips

Dips work the **lower chest** and the triceps. Dips are similar to decline press in its ability to target the lower chest. Many use dips for chest development by going deep into the dip movement to fully stretch the chest. This is a chest finishing exercise that can be substituted within the exercises listed in the *Body Part Exercise Key* for the chest, but is best alternated with decline press.

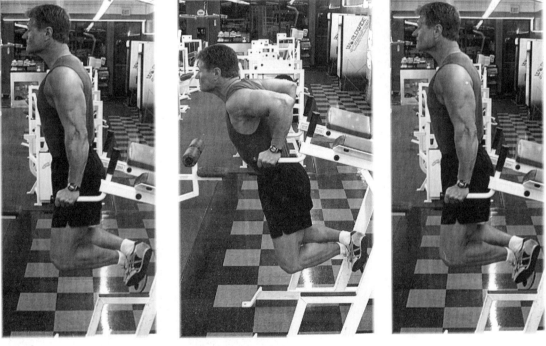

Start   Deep dip position   Up

Pullovers

Pullovers target the **ribcage area** of your chest. It generally only takes one set of 20 reps to work the ribcage area. This exercise also works the upper back. Simply lay on a bench as shown, lower a single, moderate weight dumbbell back over your head until arms are parallel with the floor as shown. Then fully stretch in the out position.

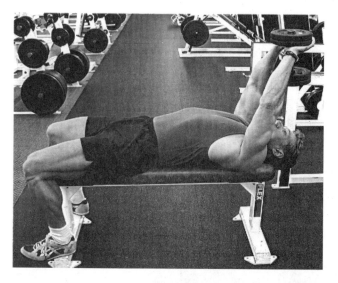

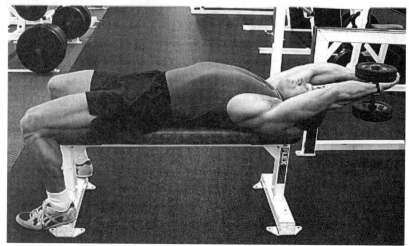

Out position–ribcage fully
stretched and extended

Up position–
dumbbell is
over forehead

Serratus Cable Pulls

The serratus muscles are located just above the ribs, slightly below the chest (pectorals) muscles on both sides. Pullovers work these muscles generally while the serratus cable pulls target these muscles directly. This exercise is somewhat difficult to perform correctly because hitting the correct areas takes some adjustment during the exercise. This exercise is good for an occasional substitution for pullovers. The key is to focus on making the serratus muscles "feel the pull" of the weight. The repetition begins with a stretched straight arm as shown. Slightly pull down and in. Your hand goes down 6 to 10 inches.

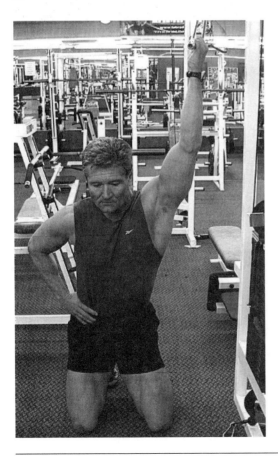 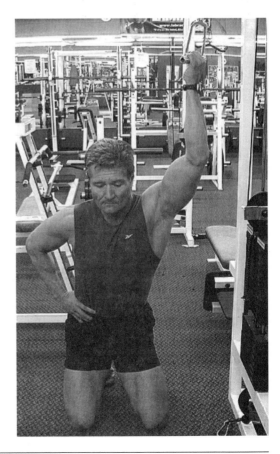

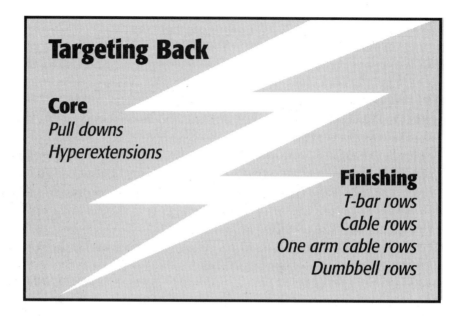

Targeting Back

Core
Pull downs
Hyperextensions

Finishing
T-bar rows
Cable rows
One arm cable rows
Dumbbell rows

Pull Downs

Pull downs target the **upper back** and can be performed by pulling the bar down in front to touch the chest or behind the neck. The behind the neck movement isolates the upper back (or lats). It is very important to make sure that you fully extend and almost stretch at the top of this exercise with front or back pull downs. Also, you should try and relax your biceps as much as possible and make your upper back do the work. Be careful not to bump your head, it's easy to do. I know from experience!

The Synergy Fitness method of Pull Downs is to combine two exercises into one. Perform the first half of the reps behind the neck, and the last half in front (as shown opposite page). The upper back muscles should fatigue during the first half of the set. By switching to front Pull Downs to finish, this increases intensity by allowing you to do more reps. And this method targets the upper-back at two different angles.

Behind the Neck Pull Downs

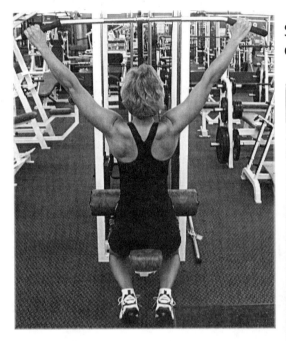

Stretch fully on
every rep

Pull down-behind neck

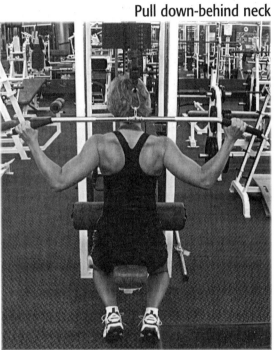

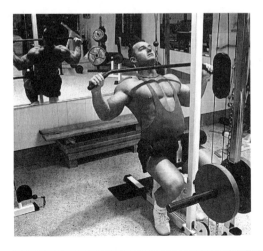

Front Pull Downs

T-Bar Rows

T-bar rows are similar to other rowing exercises targeted at the **upper back**. Start in a fully extended (stretched) position as shown, and pull the T-bar to the chest using your lats (upper-back muscles) to do the work. Careful—do not let your biceps do the work. Keep the focus on the lats.

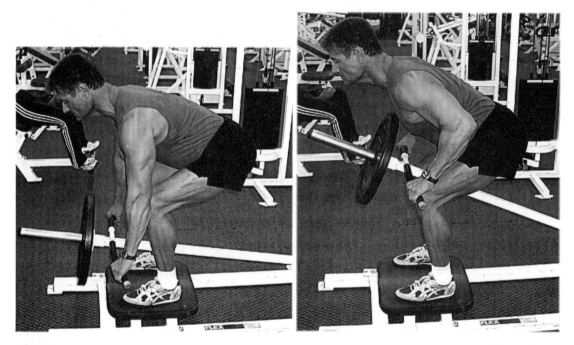

Start   Up position

Cable Rows

Cable rows receive an A+ for their ability to work the entire **upper back**. Start with your upper back straight, and fully stretched. Pull the cable toward your ribcage as shown. This exercise can also be performed with one arm for additional variation.

Start   Pull back position

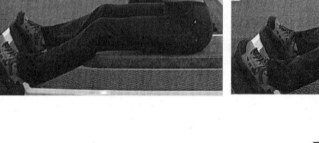

One Arm Cable Rows

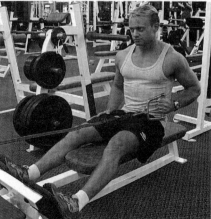

Kirk Pafford demonstrates one arm cable rows.

Dumbbell Rows

Dumbbell rows target the **upper back** and can be performed easily at home. As in all upper back exercises, fully stretch during the "down" arm extended position, and focus on not letting your biceps do the work. Correct body positioning is important to isolate upper back

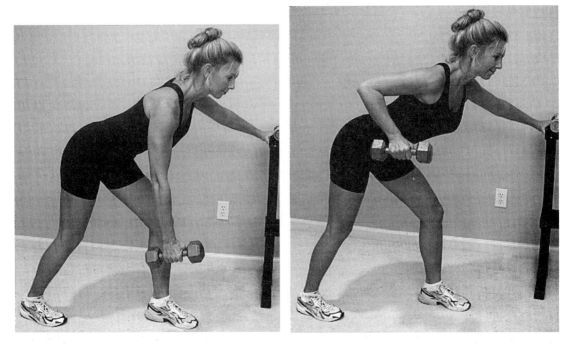

Arm extended down position   Up position

Hyperextensions

The **lower back** is the target area for hyperextensions. Go easy with this exercise and move slowly. I have injured my back with this exercise twice during my 30 years of weight training. This is a great exercise for strengthening the lower back, but you must be careful not to perform it too quickly, or jerk your body through the movement. Start this exercise with hands on your chest as shown.

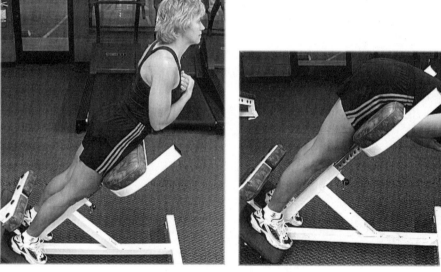

Start   Lower position

Targeting Shoulders

Core
Shoulder press
Side laterals
Shrugs

Finishing
Front laterals
Rotator cuff rotations
Rear deltoid flys or Bent laterals

Shoulder Press

Shoulder presses come in many fashions and are effective at developing the entire shoulder (deltoid) muscles. Resistance training for shoulders can prevent injury, and also injure your shoulders if the training strategy is not on target. Kate Shelby, American Classic Fitness Champ, demonstrates the dumbbell shoulder press. Dumbbells at home can provide several high quality exercises to achieve a great workout. Note for newcomers and Fitness Level One participants: the "down" position should not come down below eye level.

Down position

Press up position

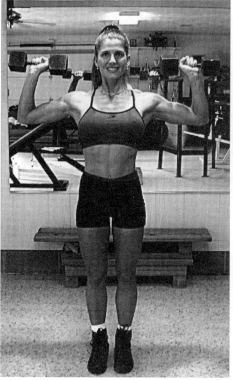
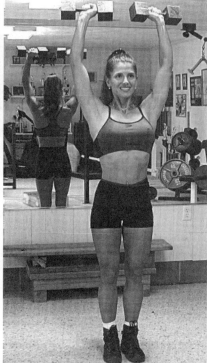

Shoulder Press

Seated barbell (behind-the-neck) shoulder press is an advanced exercise that isolates the shoulder muscles while reducing the stress in the lower back.

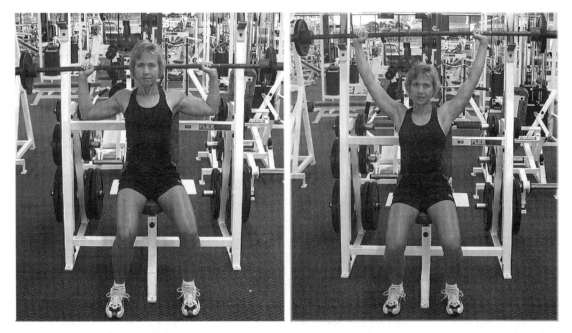

Lower bar to behind-the-neck   Press up position

The Synergy Fitness method of multi-tasking (combining) exercises to get better results faster is performed by doing half the reps behind the neck initially and the last half of the reps in front (military press) as shown (right).

Seated Shoulder Press is a variation that tends to support the lower back—especially for the advanced technique of lowering the weight to neck level. This lower position builds—but also stresses—the rotator cuff. Even at advanced levels, before going below eye level with the weights, make sure your rotator cuff is warmed-up and not tight or sore.

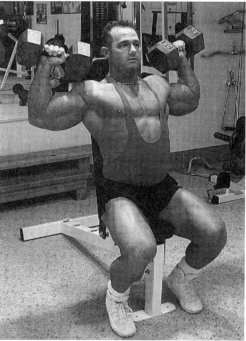

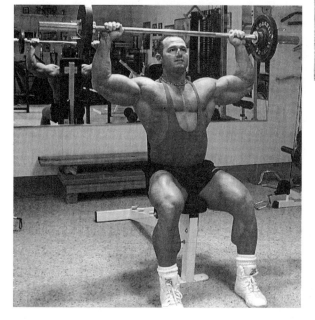

Side Laterals

Side lateral raises target the **outside center of the deltoid shoulder muscles**. Raise dumbbells from the side until you reach the up position (parallel to the floor) as shown to create maximum isolation of the muscle and less stress on the elbow. Slightly bend your elbows as the dumbbells are being raised from the side. With high-intensity training, you should feel your shoulders "burning" on the last few reps.

Start with palms in   **Raise from the side**

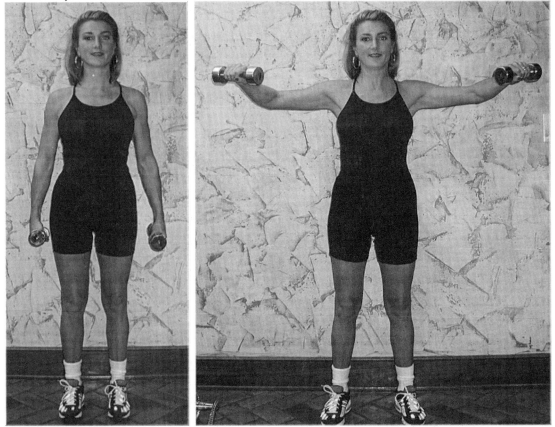

Tabitha Souder demonstrates side laterals.

Side Deltoid Twist is one variation to this exercise that may be appropriate for someone needing to spend more time developing shoulder flexibility, and strength. Without any weight initially, hold the arms out stationary—and dip the hand forward as shown (like you are pouring water into a cup) then twist the hand in the forward direction. After you learn the movement, gradually introduce light dumbbells for resistance.

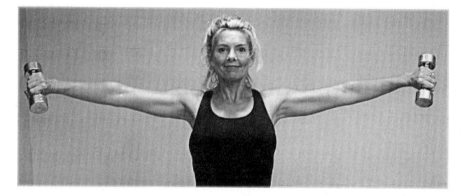

Side Deltoid Twist

Front Laterals

Front lateral raises target the **front deltoid and rotator cuff.** To reduce stress from the lower back, alternating arms and completely finish the rep with one arm before beginning with the other. And slightly bend the elbows to move the stress from the elbow joints to the shoulder deltoid muscles.

Create synergy by multi-tasking this exercise. By keeping your palms-down for the first 5–8 reps, and then finishing the set with palms-in on the last 5-8 reps—you will be performing two exercises in one.

Start

Palms down during first reps

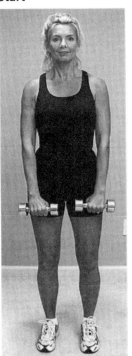
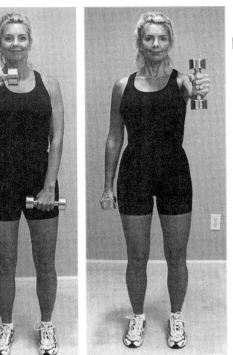

Palms in for last reps

Rotator Cuff Rotations

This exercise has an A+ rating for effectiveness. All ages should be performing this exercise. It builds strength and flexibility in the injury prone rotator cuff. This is a "must do" exercise for women, and athletes that throw. Using light weight start with the weight at your ribcage as shown. With elbow stationary and tucked into your side, slowly rotate the weight as far to the outside as possible, and return.

Start   Rotate out   Rotate in

Advanced-out position

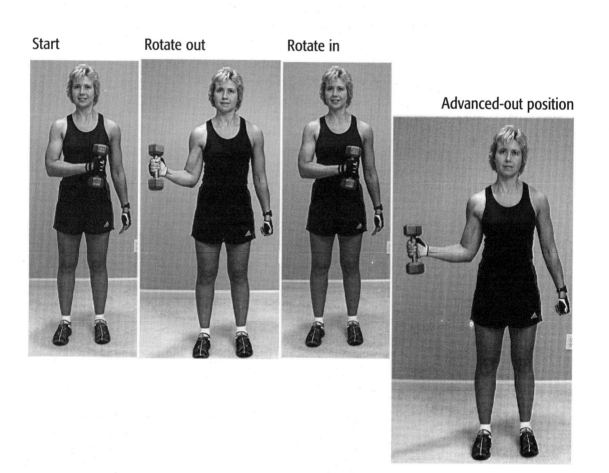

Rear Deltoid Flys

Rear Deltoid flys are typically performed on a Pec Deck or Chest Fly machine—except in reverse. There are two ways to position your hands in order to multi-task exercises. The Synergy Fitness method; perform the first half of the set with "palms in" as shown. This method fatigues the muscles quickly. For the remaining reps, turn your hands out (right) and pull the resistance backward using your rear deltoids –like the swimming breast stroke.

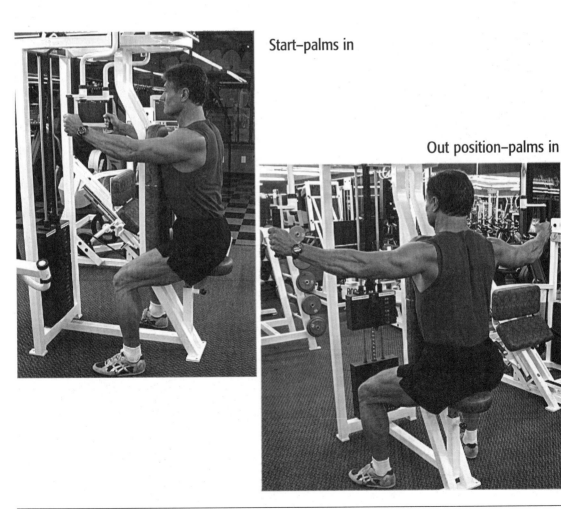

Start–palms in

Out position–palms in

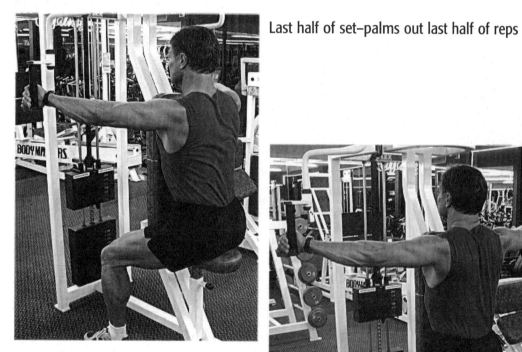

Last half of set–palms out last half of reps

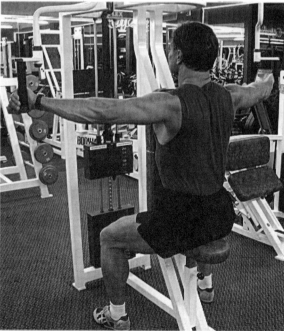

Bent Lateral Raises

Bent Lateral Raises target the **rear deltoids**. This exercise gets an A+ for its ability to strengthen the rear shoulder muscle, which are often neglected.

Start   Raise upward–palms down

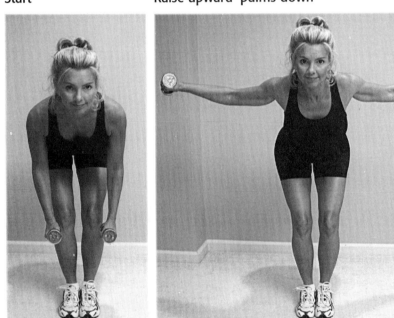

Shoulder Shrugs

Shoulders shrugs target the **traps.** Your trap muscles (trapezius) cover a large area and run from the top of your neck outward to your shoulders and about halfway down your upper back. It's true that some football players want their traps (and other muscles) to be so big that it frightens opponents. Shoulder shrugs, in moderation, will not develop your traps to this level, but shrugs will strengthen your traps.

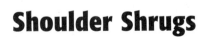

Stress likes to zap the neck and the traps. Stress makes people tighten these muscles without realizing it. End result: head aches and neck tension. Shrugs will strengthen these stress-targeted muscles.

Rotate the shoulders up and around in a forward circle for the first 10 reps. Then reverse the circle for the last 10 reps. Slightly bend the elbows and the knees during the circling motion. Some bodybuilders using heavy weight for shrugs would need to stay with the straight (up-and-down) motion, rather than the circular motion that is used with light to moderate weights.

Start   **Rotate shoulders –full in circle**

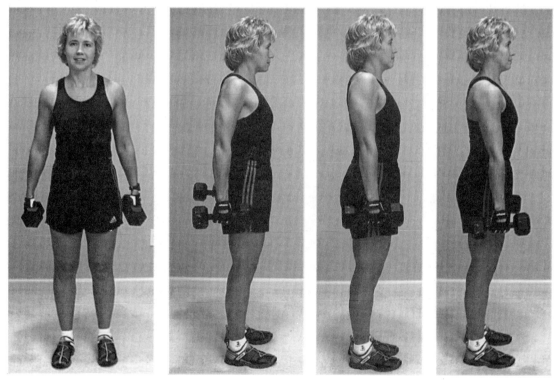

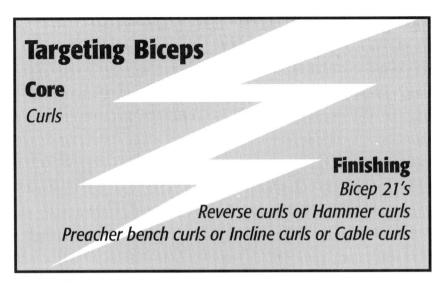

Targeting Biceps

Core
Curls

Finishing
Bicep 21's
Reverse curls or Hammer curls
Preacher bench curls or Incline curls or Cable curls

Bicep Curls

Bicep curls have taken many forms. And depending on the strategy, some methods are more effective than others. Free weight standing barbell curls are the "standard." However, dumbbells provide a great workout and reduce stress on the lower back.

Barbell curls - standing

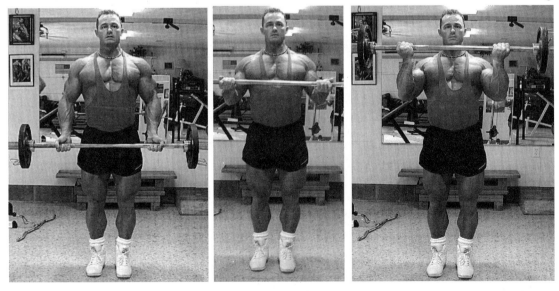

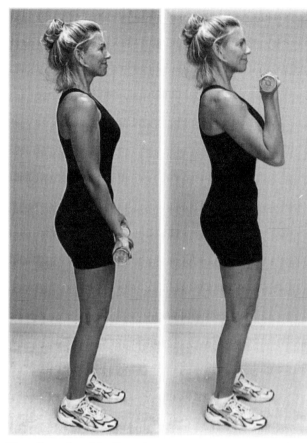

Standing dumbbell curls

Seated dumbbell curls

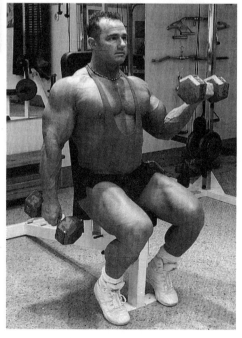

Incline Bench or
Preacher Bench Curls

Preacher bench curls are performed with the arm positioned over an incline bench. This exercise inherited the name of preacher bench curls years ago. Many machine curl units in gyms have an "incline preacher bench" feature that isolates the biceps. Note: Always extend the arms fully on the down position.

Preacher bench dumbbell curls

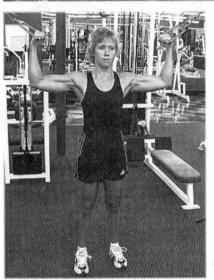

Machine curls

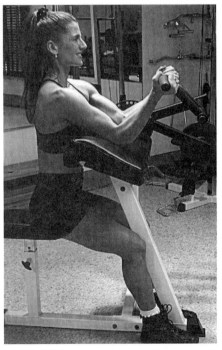

Cable curls

Concentration Curls

Concentration curls requires your concentration to position your arm to correctly isolate the biceps. Use your knee for supporting your biceps. This exercise can be performed at home. Your knee serves as the incline preacher's bench—when one is not available.

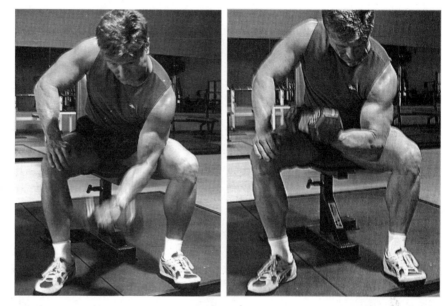

Start   Curled position

Bicep 21's

21's are my favorite bicep "finishing exercise." Keep the dumbbells in your hands for 21 total repetitions. Do 7 reps from the fully extended start position to halfway up. Follow immediately with 7 reps from the halfway point   halfway to all the way up. Then do 7 complete reps for a   total of 21 reps. This exercise will achieve the desirable "burn" in your biceps. Bicep 21's can be performed on any of the curl exercises, but the seated dumbbell curl and the concentration curl are well suited for 21's.

Hammer Curls

Hammer curls are performed with dumbbells and alternating arms. This exercise targets both the **forearms** and biceps, and is a great finishing exercise. The curl is performed with palms facing in. The two main methods are demonstrated. The dumbbell may be raised up and straight out from the body as shown by Bambi LaFont, or may be kept close to the front of the body as shown by Nick Shelby. Completely finish the rep with one arm before starting the next rep.

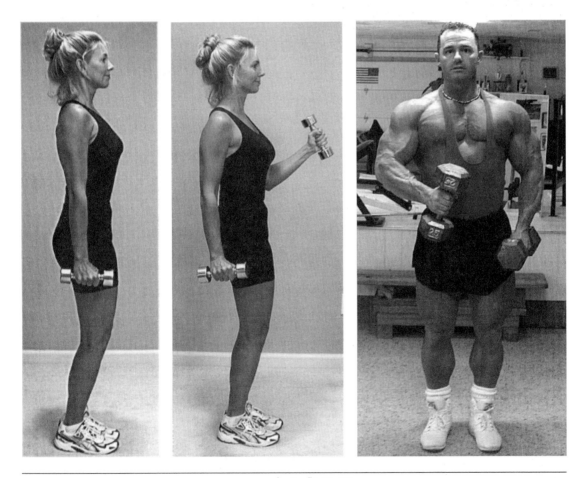

Reverse Forearm Curls

Reverse curls move the target area of curls from the biceps to the **forearms.** Reverse curls means that you simply reverse the curl palm up position to "palms down" position as shown. Reverse curls may be performed with the barbell, dumbbells, or cables. Notice the "palms in" and "elbows tucked" to the side.

Dumbbell reverse curls

Reverse curls with an
EZ curl barbell

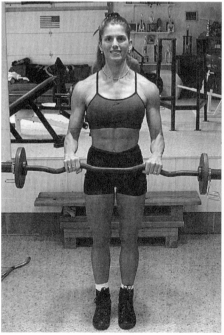

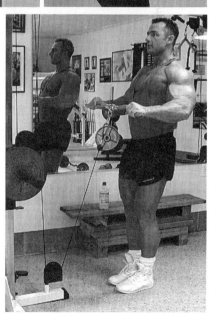

Cable
reverse curls

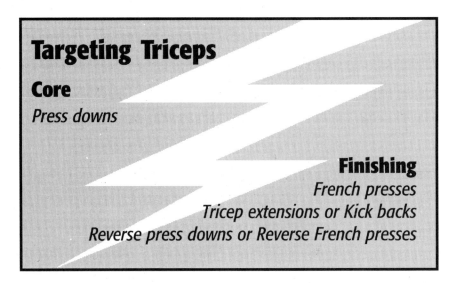

Targeting Triceps

Core
Press downs

Finishing
French presses
Tricep extensions or Kick backs
Reverse press downs or Reverse French presses

Press Downs

Tricep press downs rate an A+ for **targeting the triceps**. You can work triceps many different ways, but the press down gets great results for the entire triceps (group of 3 muscles) if performed by the principles—isolation and exhaustion with aerobic tempo between sets.

There are two parts to Synergy Fitness Press Downs. On the first 10 reps, press the rope handle downward—with an outward flair at the end of the repetition. Once your triceps are exhausted (around 10 reps) and the flair out becomes difficult, begin pumping reps straight down—with the rope handle side-by-side (last 10 reps). This method should have your triceps "burning" by 20 reps.

The rope is preferred over the bar because it creates   better isolation, and it takes stress off the elbow. Personally, I find that it takes 20 reps with moderate weight to exhaust this naturally strong group of muscles.

Triceps tend to be a problem area for women. While "spot reducing" is somewhat controversial, extra work with triceps seems to have an impact on the triceps—whereas waist spot reduction does not.

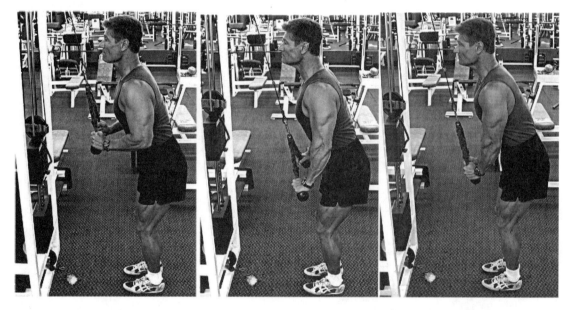

Start
Forearms parallel to floor

Extended - first 10 reps
Flair hands out at end

Pump out - last 10 reps
Hands straight down

Reverse Press Downs

Reverse Press Downs is the same exercise as Press Downs—except the hands are turned upward as shown and a bar is used rather than the rope handles. This places emphasis on the outer part of the triceps. And this is a solid "finishing" exercise.

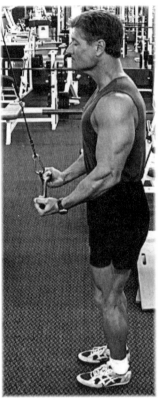

Hands
turned upward

Start   Extended

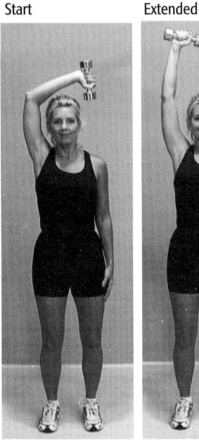

Tricep Extensions

Overhead tricep extensions offer an excellent method for effectively working triceps. Warning, watch your head as you lower the dumbbell. And using a mirror to monitor your form with this exercise is recommended.

French Presses, Nose Breaks, Skull Crushers, and Hairlines... all the Same Exercise

Thirty years ago, we called this exercise French presses. Today, the names vary, but the results are the same. This exercise is a great tricep finishing exercise. Careful with this exercise, it is definitely advanced. Why do you think someone named this exercise nose breaks, and skull crushers? Hairlines might be a good name because you lower the weight to your forehead hairline and press upward while making your triceps do the work.

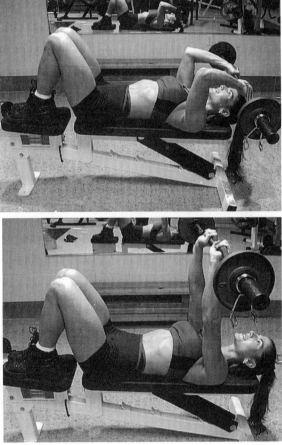

Reverse French presses. targets the outside head of the triceps.

Tricep Kickbacks

Tricep kickbacks rate an A+ as a tricep finishing exercise, and are wonderful for women wanting extra work for their triceps. Low weight and high reps will get the desirable high-intensity "burn" going. And that is the goal with this exercise!

Want results fast: Make your triceps burn during your resistance training. Careful, the tendency is to allow the shoulder to enter this exercise to assist burning triceps. Isolate the triceps by performing the exercise as shown.

Start   Extended back

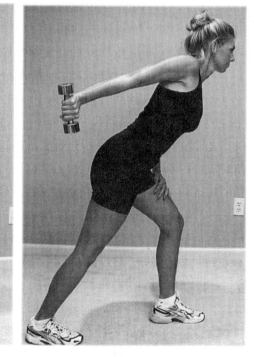

Targeting Quads

Core
Leg extensions
Leg press or Squats

Finishing
Hack squats or Front Squats
Dumbbell squats
Lunges or One leg squats

Leg Extensions

Leg extensions target the lower half of the **quads**, particularly muscles around the knees. Moderate weight and 20 repetitions will qualify as high intensity work—and lessen stress on the knees. Personally, I find that it takes 20 reps on most quad exercises to achieve "exhaustion" during every set.

Start

Full extension, up position

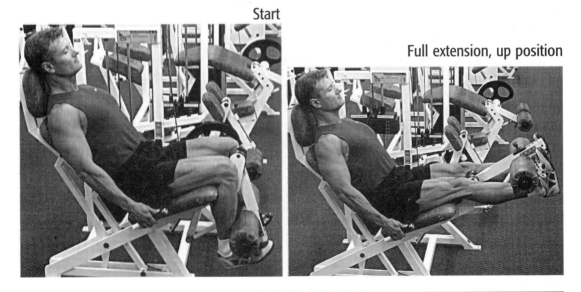

Note: If you have ACL knee problems, checking with your physician may be a good idea before adding this exercise. **Protect your knees**—ACL thinning occurs in women over the age of forty. Should you experience any pain in your knees with any resistance exercise, STOP IMMEDIATELY, and see your physician. While ACL replacement surgery is available through advances in medical science to replace torn or shattered ACL's, ACL surgery and months of painful rehab is not a good backup plan.

Squats

Squats score high as a muscle builder. Clearly, squats provide high-intensity training for overall quad development.

Start   Lower squat position

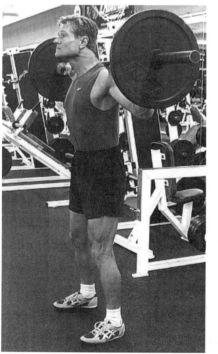 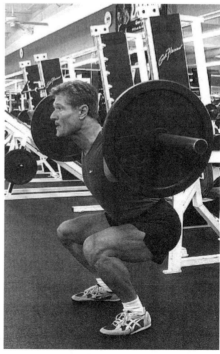

Thighs parallel
to floor
before standing

Research from Duke University Medical Center shows that deep squats that go below parallel) increases the risk of injuring knee ligaments and the meniscus, (*Knee biomechanics of the dynamic squat exercise*, Escamilla, 2001).

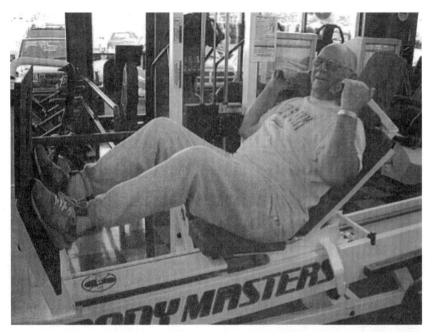

Freddie Hutchinson demonstrates leg presses.
(squat alternate)

Front Squats

Front squats are a variation of the core exercise, squats. Front squats tend to isolate the center front part of the quads. The best method is on the Smith Machine as shown. Thighs should be parallel to the floor in the squat position before returning up.

Start   Squat position

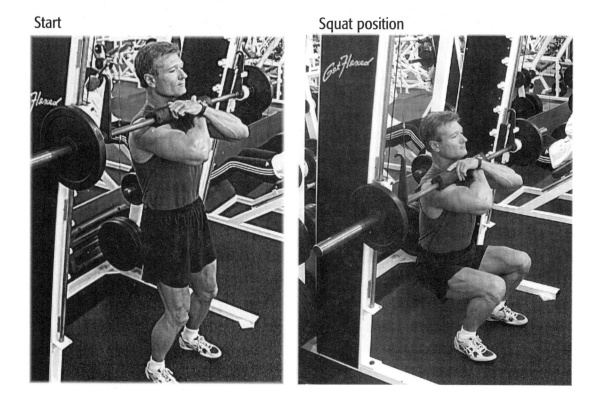

Dumbbell Squats

Dumbbell squats are easily performed at home, and perfect for Fitness Level One and newcomers to weight training.

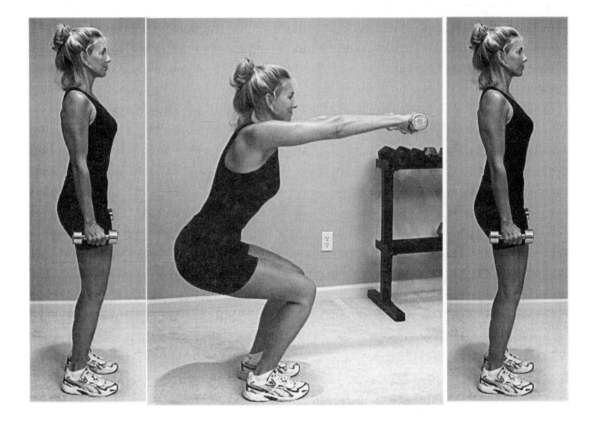

Leg Press

Leg press targets the **quads** (and the upper hamstring also gets some work). This machine allows you to increase intensity by adding moderate to heavy weight. And your back is supported with this exercise. Personally, I find that 20 reps with moderate weight produces great results. Need leg development? Try 20 reps of leg presses. Quads are strong durable muscles that will respond to high reps with moderate weight.

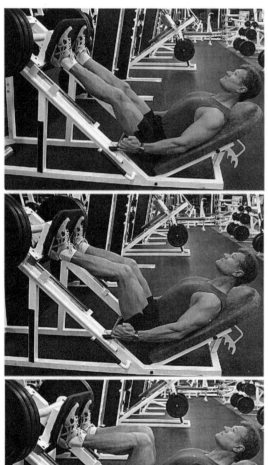

Up position

Midway position

Down position

One Leg Press

A variation on the leg press is using one leg at a time to increase isolation.

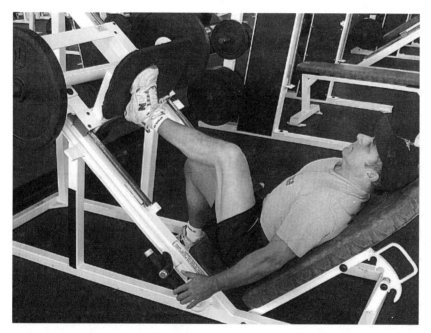

Postmaster, Bobby Allen,
demonstrates the one leg press.

Lunges

Lunges are performed during plyometric workouts (Chapter 9) and during weight training leg workouts, with dumbbells. This exercise is great for your quads (quadriceps/ thighs) upper and lower, upper-hamstrings and gluts. Lunges can be performed easily at home. If you do not have a large room or a hallway to walk down during lunges, stationary lunges also work well. Stationary lunges can be performed by returning to the original start position after every repetition.

Start   Forward lunge position

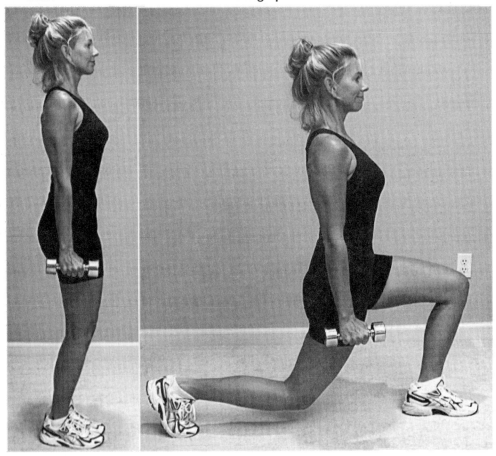

Hack Squats

Hack Squats are a favorite for developing quads. Hack squats are essentially front squats with back support. A wide stance works the inner thighs. And a close stance targets the outer quads.

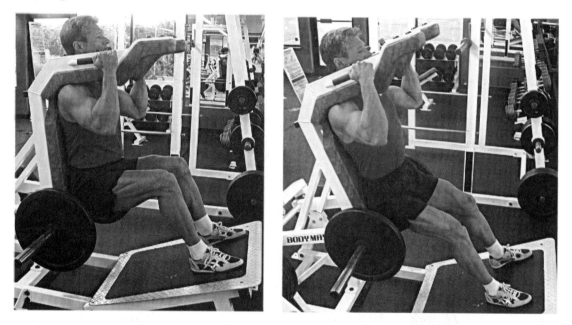

One Leg Squats

This is an advanced level exercise that is productive for developing quads and upper hamstrings necessary for sports speed development.

Start   Forward position   Advanced forward position

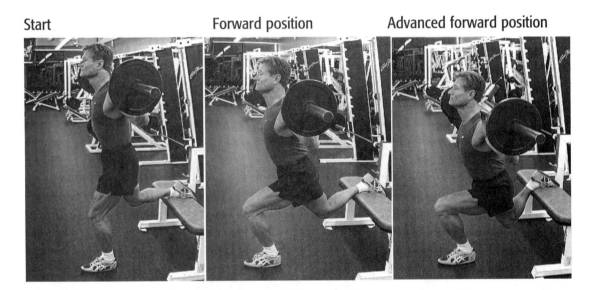

Targeting Hamstrings

Core
Leg curls

Finishing
Stiff leg dead lifts

Hamstring strength and flexibility are important in many activities from sports to injury prevention for the aging. Researchers in England demonstrate that hamstring strength and flexibility relate to low-back injury in active individuals. The researchers show that six months of hamstring strength training can contribute to a reduction in low-back injury, (*Knee flexion to extension peak torque ratios and low-back injuries in highly active individuals*, 1997, Koutedakis).

Leg Curls

Hamstring development is generally lacking in most individuals and athletes. The balance between the quads (front) and the hamstrings (rear) always favors the quads. Typically, the quads are 2 times as strong as the hamstrings. And this is not desirable. The hamstrings should be 75 to 80 percent as strong as the quads (leg extension vs. leg curl) to have the optimum balance.

Want speed? Want to improve athletic performance? The secret is here. Experts report that most athletes have hamstrings that are 50 percent as strong as the quads, (*Dintiman*, 1998). And this needs to be improved by 25 percent. Improving the flexibility and strength of your hamstrings will do more than you can imagine—no matter what your age, college athlete or grandmother—improving the strength and flexibility of your hamstrings will help you improve almost everything you do physically!

Single Leg Curls

Start

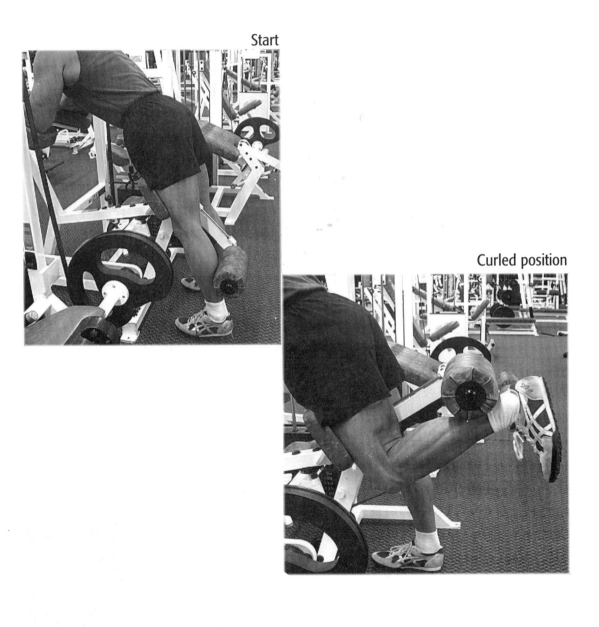

Curled position

Dumbbell Leg Curls

Like the leg curls performed on curl machines, a dumbbell and a bench at the gym or at home provides a solid hamstring exercise.

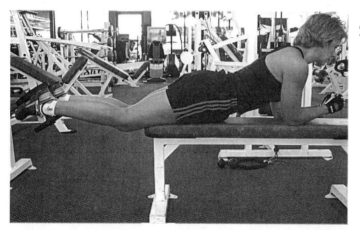
Start

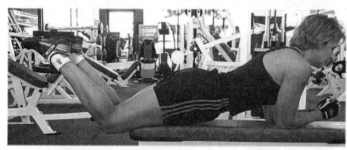
Raise weight upward

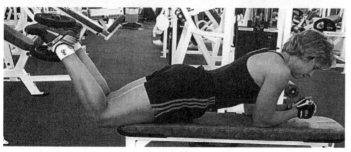
Up position, lower to repeat

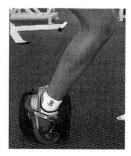

The trick to this exercise is placing the dumbbell between your feet (right) and carefully hanging your knees off the bench approximately 4" to begin the exercise.

Stiff Leg Dead Lifts

The lower back and upper hamstrings receive the greatest benefit from stiff leg dead lifts. Only don't keep your knees perfectly straight. The name is "stiff leg," but slightly bend your knees and stop just past midway (as shown) until you are ready to move to more advanced levels.

Start

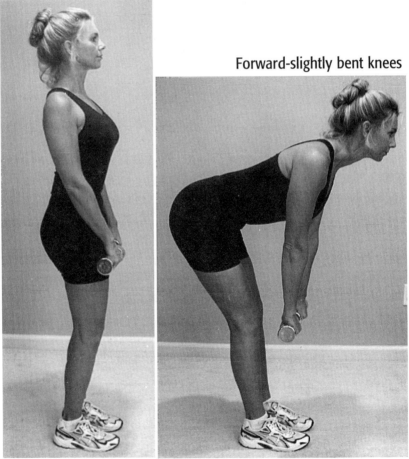

Forward-slightly bent knees

This position stretches hamstrings significantly. Since the upper part of the hamstrings is the typically the weakest point, make sure you have been stretching for 60 days before performing this advanced position.

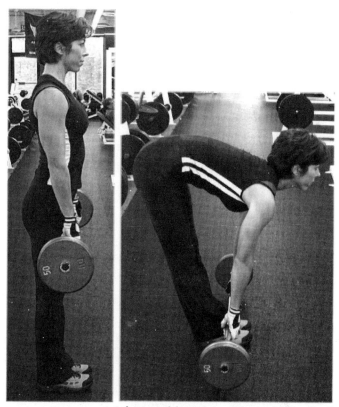

Advanced-lower position with barbell

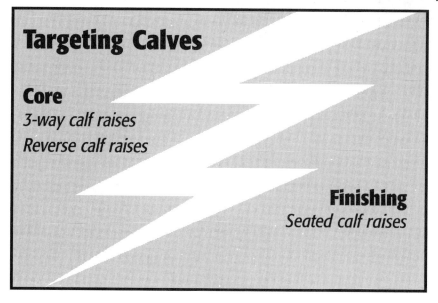

Targeting Calves

Core
3-way calf raises
Reverse calf raises

Finishing
Seated calf raises

3-Way Calf Raises

Calf raises can be performed on a gym machine as shown or at home on a step. Calves are durable muscles that take more reps to achieve exhaustion (at least 20 reps per set).

The Synergy Fitness method targets all angles of your calves by performing the sets and reps by equal number in three directions (shown right). Example: If your Strategic Fitness Plan calls for 3 sets, then perform each set with your toes pointed in three different directions on different sets. If your Fitness Plan calls for 1 set of 21, then change positions every 7 reps.

**At home
just need a step**

Fully stretch between reps

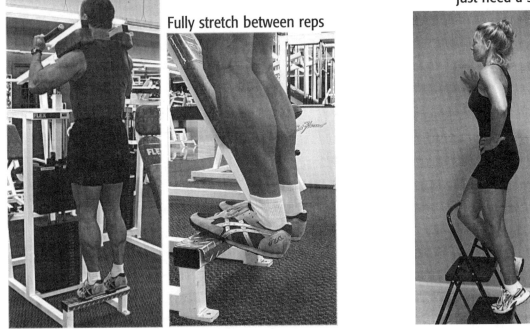

Gym
calf raise
machine

Important: To isolate calf muscles, it is essential to go down as far as possible and fully stretch your calves and achilles tendons during every rep as shown. Don't count the rep unless your heels go all the way down.

3 Way Calf Raises

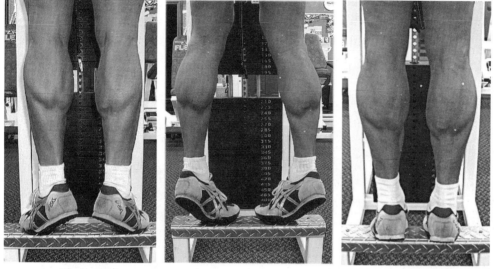

Toes out   In   Straight

Reverse Calf Raises

Placing your bodyweight on your heels and hanging both feet off the front of a step, as shown, positions you for reverse calf raises. Keep knees straight.

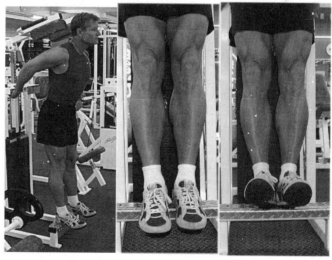

Heals on step   Down   Up

Seated Calf Raises

Seated calf raises hit the calves in a slightly different angle than standing calf raises. This exercise serves well as a finishing exercise.

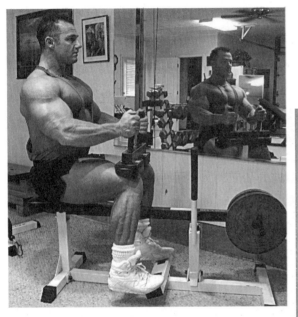

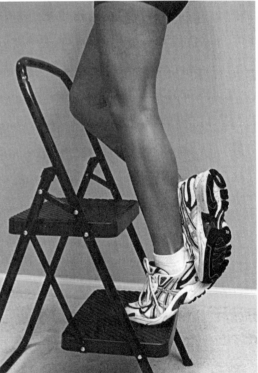

Calf Raises at Home

Calf raises can be performed with the resistance of your bodyweight—especially if you use one leg at a time as shown. All you need is a step.

Stubborn Calves?
Try the Sprint 8 Workout

The **Sprint 8 Workout** (*Chapter 8*) will develop calves, hamstrings and quads, unlike any other exercise. Bodybuilders with stubborn calf muscles might consider experimenting with sprinting and bleacher running to supplement weight training for calf and hamstring development.

Personally, I only do 3-way calf raises (3 sets of 20 reps) once a week along with the Sprint 8 Workouts (and no special dieting). Typical weight training primarily hits the slow twitch muscles. Calves are responsive when all three muscle fiber types are worked (Chapter 4).

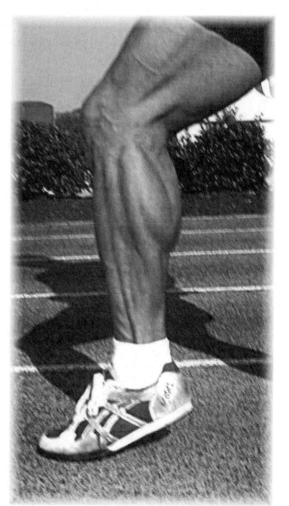

The Target Zone Training Method suggests that you target slow-twitch calf muscles with traditional calf raises, and target fast-twitch fibers with the Sprint 8 Workout.

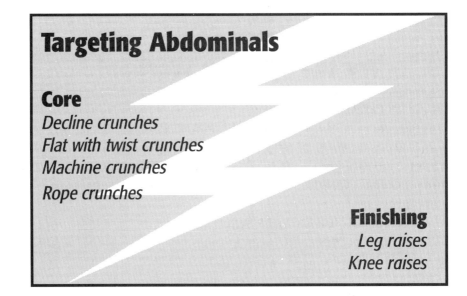

Targeting Abdominals

Core
Decline crunches
Flat with twist crunches
Machine crunches
Rope crunches

Finishing
Leg raises
Knee raises

Decline Crunches

Crunches resemble quarter sit-ups and target the abs. Start in a fully expanded (ribs out) position, and roll your shoulders forward to crunch your abs. Keep your lower back touching the bench and raise your upper back off the bench by around six inches. Some call this exercise "cramp" sit-ups. Good name, because this exercise sets your abs on fire. Decline bench crunches get an A+ for adding intensity to the exercise.

Fully stretched—Back position

Up position

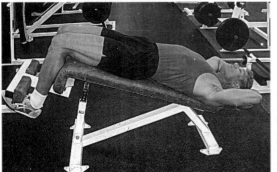
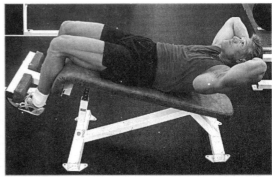

When you feel the "burning" in the abs, that's the beginning of high-intensity training. The test is—how many reps you do after the burning starts. When the abs begin to burn and I think I can't do any more, I quit thinking...and try to block out the pain for 5 to 10 more reps.

It's a wise strategy to change the method of crunches every 30 days. Several alternate methods follow.

Crunches

Crunches (sometimes called flat, mat, or floor crunches) are the basic exercise for the **abs**. Crunches have replaced sit-ups because the sit-up places stress on the lower back—rather the abs. Crunches isolate the abs for high-intensity training and superior results.

Crunches up position

Crunches with twist

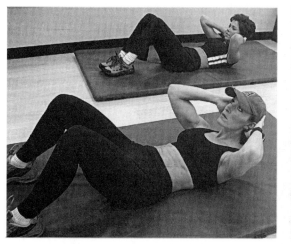
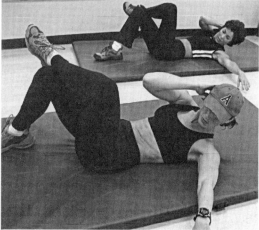

Machine Crunches

Machines for crunches are made by most resistance training equipment manufacturers, and various abdominal machines are usually available in most gyms. While the ab machines seem to copy the basic floor crunch, some machines hit the abs in different ways making them a solid selection.

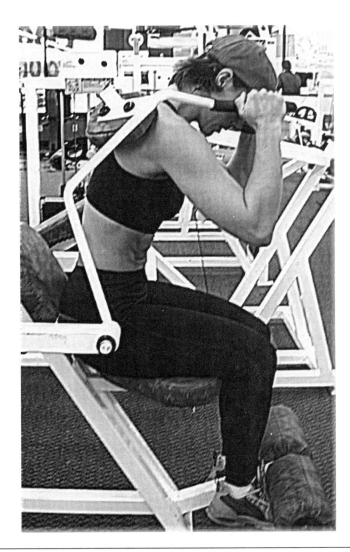

Rope Crunches

Crunches, using a cable (with the rope handles places high-intensity on the **abs** (and some stress on the lower back). This is a great exercise, but use caution and monitor your lower back.

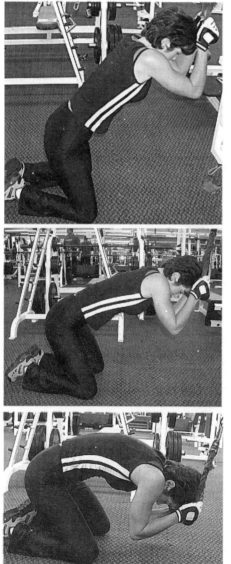

Start position
–rope in hands

Pull toward floor

Fully crunched position

Leg Raises

Leg raises target the **lower abs** and hip flexors. Perform the flat, or floor leg raises.

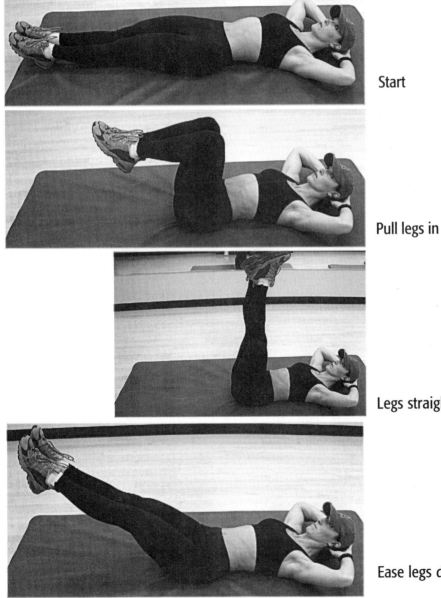

Start

Pull legs in

Legs straight up

Ease legs down slowly

Machine Leg Raises

Leg raises on the standing leg raise unit is a favorite for targeting the **abs** while reducing stress from the lower back. These are performed like the flat leg raises except you are leaning on the back of the unit (rather than the floor or a bench) in an upright, hanging position.

Start

Raise-with bent knees

Advanced – legs straight

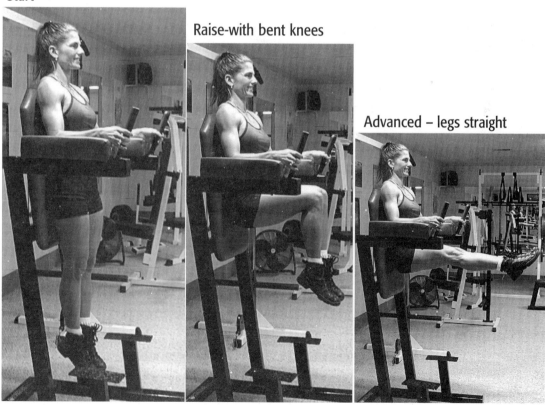

Seated Knee Raises

Seated knee raises offer a substitute for leg raises. Knee raises work the **lower abs** and can be done from the floor or on a bench.

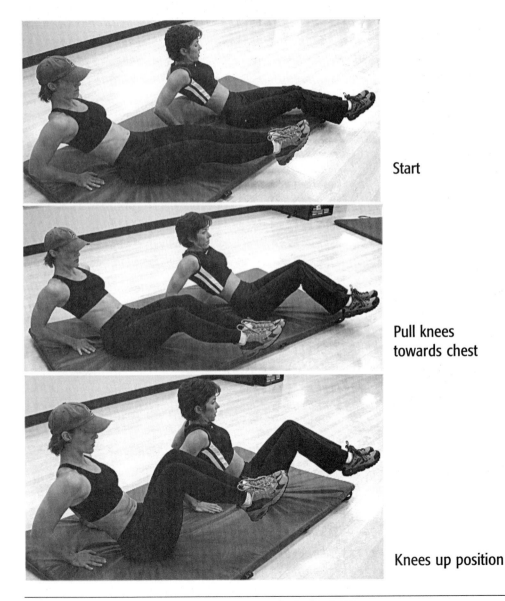

Start

Pull knees
towards chest

Knees up position

Targeting Obliques

Core
Side bends

Twists

Finishing
Balanced diet in moderation

Side Bends

Side bends offer a quick and easy way to work obliques and increase flexibility in the lower back. The all time best developer of obliques is a balanced diet in moderation.

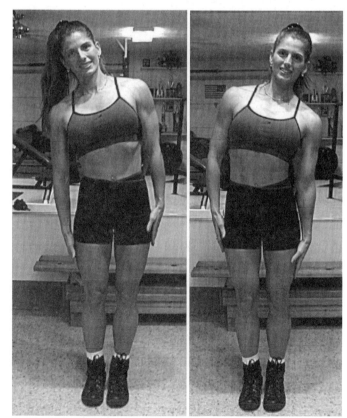

Twists

Twists seem simple, but this is a solid exercise for your obliques and lower back. This is a light exercise performed without weights because conventional thinking is that you do not want heavy exercises for obliques.

Arms up and twist from side to side

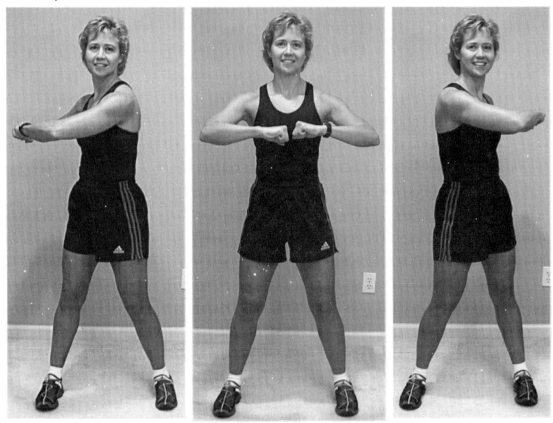

Conclusion

You have successfully completed the "Set" phase and now it's time to begin the "GO" phase by following a Strategic Fitness Plan in the next chapter. All exercises listed in the Strategic Fitness Plans have been illustrated, and major components of Synergy Fitness have been discussed. Your Strategic Fitness Plan comes together in the following chapter and it's time to begin Synergy Fitness Training.

11

Strategic Fitness Plans

Ready, set, GO! Its time to implement the GO phase!

You have successfully competed the **Ready** section (Chapters 1–4) by learning **about Synergy Fitness**—how to increase growth hormone naturally; and target your three types of muscle fiber and three energy systems that will tone and build muscle, and turn your body into a fat eating machine.

You have successfully completed the **Set** section (Chapters 5–9) by obtaining specific technical knowledge about the five major components of Synergy Fitness. You have learned how to multi-task exercises for timesaving efficiency; how to implement the individual components of Synergy Fitness; and you have discovered the Fitness Level that is appropriate for you as you begin your fitness plan.

Now, it's time to jump-start the **GO** phase and begin receiving all the fantastic benefits Synergy Fitness training has to offer.

The GO Phase

This chapter outlines the GO phase of Synergy Fitness. This is an individualized exercise prescription, customized for age, training experience, and current fitness level.

Use this chapter as a workbook by charting the number of sets, reps, and weights used during training. It's important to record notes concerning your training successes. By recording notes–during, and at the completion of your workout–you can track your fitness improvement accomplishments, and set training benchmarks for the next workout.

Purchasers of this book may, for personal use, copy Strategic Fitness Plans in this chapter. Additional Training Logs are also available at www.readysetgofitness.com.

High-intensity fitness training is tough. And motivation to continue training will generally depend on seeing positive outcomes. Stick with your plan—daily and weekly—and you will see positive results every week.

Work the plan, and record your results. Research shows charting training results will yield greater success. The time you to take to chart your progress will actually save you time.

Review Your Fitness Plan Before Every Workout

Before every workout, take 5 minutes to review your previous performance, and think through the workout for the day.

Your Strategic Fitness Plan is designed to attack one day, and one week at a time. A good fitness strategy is to take a few minutes on Sunday and think through your weekly training plan. I cannot overemphasize taking 5 minutes before every workout to review your plan for the day. This five minute planning period will save you more time during the workout.

You are on your way to improved fitness, strength, appearance, and energy with every week of training. Use proven planning principles: plan your work, and then work your plan. And track your results—it will keep you focused and moving forward.

Fitness Training Levels

When in doubt start with a lower Fitness Level, you can always raise the Level at any point. The five Fitness Levels are presented in Chapter 5, *Building the Strategic Fitness Plan*. As you determine your beginning fitness training level—double-check which of the five Levels is right for you.

Carefully review discussions concerning your age, training experience, and current fitness status. The review will insure you begin at the correct fitness training level.

Level One is for newcomers to high-intensity training, adults over age 60, and children under age 14. Do not be misled; Level One is not a pushover program. It's demanding.

Level Two is for adults who have been exercising, but not with comprehensive training methods or with high-intensity workouts; and adults age 40 to 70. There is some overlapping with ages due to variables in fitness levels at various ages.

Levels Three - Five are for physically fit individuals with fitness training experience. These Levels include a split body routine for weight training (it is called "split body" because body parts are split and worked on different days). As your fitness status improves, you will become more advanced in training. And training intensity must increase to continue providing growth hormone release benchmark opportunities.

Raising the Intensity Bar

With all aspects of fitness—strength, flexibility, aerobic, power, and anaerobic capacity—you will notice improvement quickly as you follow your Strategic Fitness Plan. To keep the results coming, you need to continually keep bumping up intensity.

Gradually bumping up intensity in your strength training means you will need to gradually increase resistance every few weeks—handling more weight, sets, and reps. It may mean switching from a total body workout (Levels One and Two) to a split body routine (Levels Three through Five) in a year or so.

Increasing the intensity level in flexibility means going just a little closer to the knee during the hold position of the hurdle stretch. And, this is intense!

Bumping up intensity in anaerobic sprinting typically means beginning with two to four sprints the first week and working up to eight by the fourth week. After adding all eight sprints of the Sprint 8 Workout, intensity is increased by increasing the pace—go faster and harder, not longer.

The same holds true for increasing intensity with the aerobic and power components of Synergy Fitness—go faster and harder, not longer.

Measuring Performance of Your Strategic Fitness Plan

During your workout record the number of sets, reps, and weight used. And make notes in the appropriate grey boxes in the **Strategic Fitness Plan Training Log.**

Example: when you finish 20 minutes of cardio, write "Cardio-20" or "20 mins" in the grey box under the day of the week.

If you miss a day, use your **make up day** on Wednesday to replace this workout. Tracking your progress is critically important during the first eight-weeks of the program, but it remains important for continued success even after the initial eight-week period.

Training Logs for the first four weeks (for all five Fitness Levels) have been provided on the following pages. Before you begin, make copies of all four weeks. You will need these during the weeks following the initial training period.

Once the copies are made (these copies are for the second four week period), begin recording results on your very first workout—directly into the book.

This will provide added motivation as you go back and review your Synergy Fitness starting point. Keep these records as a reminder of how far you have progressed. See page 100 in Chapter 5 for detailed instructions for completing the Training Log.

STRATEGIC FITNESS PLAN

Exercise Prescription - Level One

MONDAY	TUESDAY	WEDNESDAY	THURSDAY	FRIDAY	SATURDAY	SUNDAY
10-Minute Stretching Routine *Chapter 6*	**Weights** 30 minutes *Chapter 10*	**10-Minute Stretching Routine**	**Weights** 30 minutes	**10-Minute Stretching Routine**	**10-Minute Stretching Routine**	Rest
Sprint 8 20 minutes *Chapter 8*	**Cardio-20** 20 minutes *Chapter 7*	Make up day	**Cardio-20** 20 minutes	**Sprint 8**	**Cardio-20** or **Weights**	
						TOTAL WEEK TIME: 3 hours 20 mins
30 minutes	50 minutes	10 minutes	50 minutes	30 minutes	30 minutes	

STRATEGIC FITNESS PLAN								
Training Log Level One Week 1 Date_____								

Workout:	Training Plan:		M	T	W	Th	F	Sat	S
10-Minute Stretching	**3 x week (M, W, F, Sat)** *Chapter 6*		▓		▓		▓	▓	
Cardio *Chapter 7*	**30 minutes 2 x week** *Tuesday, Thursday or Saturday*			▓		▓		▓	
Sprint 8 *Chapter 8*	**20 minutes 2 x week** *20-40% speed/intensity during first 4 weeks. 8 reps 70-yards, walk back.*		▓				▓		
Plyometrics *Chapter 9*	*Plyometric drills begin at Level Two*								

Weight Training:	Exercise: *Chapter 10*		**Record Sets & Reps** *Performance* sets /reps	*Record amount of weight used during sets in shaded areas.* **NOTE: Perform Weight-plyo techniques** *(Chapter 9)* **on first 3 to 5 reps per set.**					
Chest	Bench press	1/12	▓	▓	▓	▓	▓	▓	
	Incline press	1/12	▓						
	Chest stretch	30 sec	▓						
Back	Pull downs	1/12	▓	▓	▓	▓	▓	▓	
	Up back stretch	30 sec	▓						
Shoulders	Shoulder press	1/10	▓	▓	▓	▓	▓	▓	
	Shrugs	1/15	▓						
	Shoulder stretch	30 sec	▓						
	Rotator cuff	1/10	▓						
Biceps	Curls	1/10	▓	▓	▓	▓	▓	▓	
	Incline DB curl	1/10	▓						
Triceps	Press downs	1/20	▓	▓	▓	▓	▓	▓	
Quads	Leg ext	1/20	▓	▓	▓	▓	▓	▓	
Hamstrings	Leg curls	1/12	▓	▓	▓	▓	▓	▓	
Calves	3-way calf raises	1/21	▓	▓	▓	▓	▓	▓	
Abs	Crunches	1/15	▓	▓	▓	▓	▓	▓	
Obliques	Twists	1/15	▓	▓	▓	▓	▓	▓	

STRATEGIC FITNESS PLAN

Training Log   Level One   Week 2   Date_____

Workout:	Training Plan:		M	T	W	Th	F	Sat	S
10-Minute Stretching	**3 x week (M, W, F, Sat)** *Chapter 6*		▓		▓		▓	▓	
Cardio *Chapter 7*	**30 minutes 2 x week** *Tuesday, Thursday or Saturday*			▓		▓		▓	
Sprint 8 *Chapter 8*	**20 minutes 2 x week** *20-40% speed/intensity* *during first 4 weeks. 8 reps 70-yards, walk back.*		▓			▓			
Plyometrics *Chapter 9*	*Plyometric drills* *begin at Level Two*								

Weight Training:	**Exercise:** *Chapter 10*	**Record Sets & Reps** ***Performance*** *sets /reps*	*Record amount of weight used during sets in shaded areas.* ***NOTE: Perform Weight-plyo techniques*** *(Chapter 9)* ***on first 3 to 5 reps per set.***						
Chest	Bench press 1/12 Incline press 1/12 Chest stretch 30 sec	▓▓▓▓	▓	▓	▓	▓	▓	▓	
Back	Pull downs 1/12 Up back stretch 30 sec	▓▓▓	▓	▓	▓	▓	▓	▓	
Shoulders	Shoulder press 1/10 Shrugs 1/15 Shoulder stretch 30 sec Rotator cuff 1/10	▓▓▓▓	▓	▓	▓	▓	▓	▓	
Biceps	Curls 1/10 Incline DB curl 1/10	▓▓▓	▓	▓	▓	▓	▓	▓	
Triceps	Press downs 1/20	▓	▓	▓	▓	▓	▓	▓	
Quads	Leg press 1/20	▓	▓	▓	▓	▓	▓	▓	
Hamstrings	Leg curls 1/12	▓	▓	▓	▓	▓	▓	▓	
Calves	3-way calf raises 1/21	▓	▓	▓	▓	▓	▓	▓	
Abs	Crunches 1/15	▓	▓	▓	▓	▓	▓	▓	
Obliques	Side bends 1/15	▓	▓	▓	▓	▓	▓	▓	

STRATEGIC FITNESS PLAN

Training Log　　Level One　　Week 3　　Date_____

Workout:	Training Plan:		M	T	W	Th	F	Sat	S
10-Minute Stretching	**3 x week (M, W, F, Sat)** *Chapter 6*		▓		▓		▓	▓	
Cardio *Chapter 7*	**30 minutes 2 x week** *Tuesday, Thursday or Saturday*			▓		▓		▓	
Sprint 8 *Chapter 8*	**20 minutes 2 x week** *20-40% speed/intensity during first 4 weeks. 8 reps 70-yards, walk back.*			▓		▓		▓	
Plyometrics *Chapter 9*	***Plyometric drills begin at Level Two***								
Weight Training:	**Exercise:** *Chapter 10*	**Record Sets & Reps** *Performance* *sets/reps*	*Record amount of weight used during sets in shaded areas.* ***NOTE: Perform Weight-plyo techniques*** *(Chapter 9)* ***on first 3 to 5 reps per set.***						
Chest	Bench press　　　1/12	_____							
	Incline press　　　1/12	_____							
	Chest stretch　　30 sec	_____							
Back	Pull downs　　　1/12	_____							
	Up back stretch　30 sec	_____							
Shoulders	Shoulder press　　1/10	_____							
	Shrugs　　　　　1/15	_____							
	Shoulder stretch　30 sec	_____							
	Rotator cuff　　　1/10	_____							
Biceps	Curls　　　　　　1/10	_____							
	Incline DB curl　　1/10	_____							
Triceps	Press downs　　　1/20								
Quads	Leg ext　　　　　1/20								
Hamstrings	Leg curls　　　　1/12								
Calves	3-way calf raises　1/21								
Abs	Crunches　　　　1/15								
Obliques	Twists　　　　　1/15								

STRATEGIC FITNESS PLAN

Training Log   Level One   Week 4   Date_____

Workout:	Training Plan:		M	Tu	W	Th	F	Sat	S
10-Minute Stretching	**3 x week (M, W, F, Sat)** *Chapter 6*		▓		▓		▓	▓	
Cardio *Chapter 7*	**30 minutes 1 x week** *Tuesday, Thursday or Saturday*			▓		▓		▓	
Sprint 8 *Chapter 8*	**20 minutes 2 x week** *20-40% speed/intensity during first 4 weeks. 8 reps 70-yards, walk back.*			▓			▓		
Plyometrics *Chapter 9*	*Plyometric drills begin at Level Two*								
Weight Training:	**Exercise:** *Chapter 10*	**Record Sets & Reps Performance** *sets/reps*	*Record amount of weight used during sets in shaded areas.* ***NOTE: Perform Weight-plyo techniques*** *(Chapter 9)* ***on first 3 to 5 reps per set.***					

Weight Training	Exercise	sets/reps	M	Tu	W	Th	F	Sat	S
Chest	Bench press	1/12	▓	▓	▓	▓	▓	▓	
	Incline press	1/12	▓						
	Chest stretch	30 sec	▓						
Back	Pull downs	1/12	▓	▓	▓	▓	▓	▓	
	Up back stretch	30 sec	▓						
Shoulders	Shoulder press	1/10	▓	▓	▓	▓	▓	▓	
	Shrugs	1/15	▓						
	Shoulder stretch	30 sec	▓						
	Rotator cuff	1/10	▓						
Biceps	Curls	1/10	▓	▓	▓	▓	▓	▓	
	Incline DB curl	1/10	▓						
Triceps	Press downs	1/20	▓	▓	▓	▓	▓	▓	
Quads	Leg press	1/20	▓	▓	▓	▓	▓	▓	
Hamstrings	Leg curls	1/12	▓	▓	▓	▓	▓	▓	
Calves	3-way calf raises	1/21	▓	▓	▓	▓	▓	▓	
Abs	Crunches	1/15	▓	▓	▓	▓	▓	▓	
Obliques	Side bends	1/15	▓	▓	▓	▓	▓	▓	

NOTES:

NOTE: Continue the Fitness Plan for this Level until you complete your initial Eight-Week Commitment. For program continuation, additional copies of the Strategic Fitness Plans may be obtained from www.readysetgofitness.com. All purchasers of this book have permission to copy plans for personal use. After the initial eight weeks of training, repeat the Fitness Level adding intensity (more weight, reps, speed), or move to the next Fitness Level.

STRATEGIC FITNESS PLAN

Exercise Prescription - Level Two

MONDAY	TUESDAY	WEDNESDAY	THURSDAY	FRIDAY	SATURDAY	SUNDAY
10-Minute Stretching Routine *Chapter 6*	**Weights** 1 hour *Chapter 10*		**10-Minute Stretching Routine**	**10-Minute Stretching Routine**	**Weights** 1 hour	Rest
Sprint 8 20 minutes *Chapter 8*	**Cardio-20** 20 minutes *Chapter 7*	*Make up day*	**Weights** 1 hour	**Sprint 8**		
				Plyometrics *Chapter 9*		**TOTAL WEEK TIME:** 4 hours
30 minutes	1 hour 20 minutes		1 hour 10 minutes	45 minutes	1 hour	45 mins

STRATEGIC FITNESS PLAN

Training Log   Level Two   Week 1   Date_____

Workout:	Training Plan:		M	T	W	Th	F	Sat	S
10-Minute Stretching	**3 x week (M, Th, F)** *Chapter 6*		▓			▓	▓		
Cardio *Chapter 7*	**30 minutes 1 x week** *Tuesday or Thursday*			▓					
Sprint 8 *Chapter 8*	**20 minutes 2 x week** *30-50% speed/intensity during first 4 weeks. 8 reps 70-yards, walk back.*		▓				▓		
Plyometrics *Chapter 9*	**15 minutes 1 x week** *1 set plyo-drills at half-speed*		▓						

Weight Training:	Exercise: *Chapter 10*	Record Sets & Reps Performance *sets/reps*	Record amount of weight used during sets in shaded areas. ***NOTE: Perform Weight-plyo techniques (Chapter 9) on first 3 to 5 reps per set.***						
Chest	Bench press 2/12	_____							
	Incline press 1/12	_____							
	Chest stretch 30 sec	_____							
Back	Pull downs 2/12	_____							
	Up back stretch 30 sec								
Shoulders	Shoulder press 2/10	_____							
	Front laterals 1/10	_____							
	Shrugs 1/20	_____							
	Shoulder stretch 30 sec	_____							
	Rotator cuff 1/15	_____							
Biceps	Curls 2/10	_____							
	Incline DB curl 1/10	_____							
Triceps	Press downs 3/20								
Quads	Leg press 2/20	_____							
	Leg ext 1/20								
Hamstrings	Leg curls 1/15								
Calves	3-way calf raises 1/21								
Abs	Leg raises 1/20	_____							
	Crunches 1/25								
Obliques	Twists 1/20								

STRATEGIC FITNESS PLAN

Training Log   Level Two   Week 2   Date_____

Workout:	Training Plan:		M	TU	W	TH	F	SAT	S
10-Minute Stretching	**3 x week (M, Th, F)** *Chapter 6*		▓			▓	▓		
Cardio *Chapter 7*	**30 minutes 1 x week** *Tuesday or Thursday*			▓		▓			
Sprint 8 *Chapter 8*	**20 minutes 2 x week** *30-50% speed/intensity* *during first 4 weeks. 8 reps 70-yards*		▓			▓		▓	
Plyometrics *Chapter 9*	**15 minutes 1 x week** *1 set plyo-drills at half-speed*			▓			▓		
Weight Training:	**Exercise:** *Chapter 10*	**Record Sets & Reps Performance** *sets/reps*	*Record amount of weight used during sets in shaded areas.* ***NOTE: Perform Weight-plyo techniques*** *(Chapter 9)* ***on first 3 to 5 reps per set.***						
Chest	Bench press 2/12 Chest flys 1/12 Chest stretch 30 sec	_____ _____							
Back	Pull downs 2/12 Up back stretch 30 sec	_____							
Shoulders	Shoulder press 2/10 Side laterals 1/10 Shrugs 1/20 Shoulder stretch 30 sec	_____ _____ _____							
Biceps	Curls 2/10 Bicep 21's 1/10	_____							
Triceps	Press downs 2/20 Kick backs 1/12	_____							
Quads	Hack squats 2/20 Leg ext 1/20	_____							
Hamstrings	Leg curls 1/15								
Calves	3-way calf raises 1/21 Rev calf raises 1/20	_____							
Abs	Crunches 2/25								
Obliques	Side bends 1/20								

STRATEGIC FITNESS PLAN

Training Log   Level Two   Week 3   Date_____

Workout:	Training Plan:		M	T	W	Th	F	Sat	S
10-Minute Stretching	**3 x week (M, Th, F)** *Chapter 6*		▓			▓	▓		
Cardio *Chapter 7*	**30 minutes 1 x week** *Tuesday or Thursday*			▓		▓			
Sprint 8 *Chapter 8*	**20 minutes 2 x week** *30-50% speed/intensity during first 4 weeks. 8 reps 70-yards, walk back.*			▓			▓		
Plyometrics *Chapter 9*	**15 minutes 1 x week** *1 set plyo-drills*			▓					
Weight Training:	**Exercise:** *Chapter 10*	**Record Sets & Reps Performance** *sets/reps*	*Record amount of weight used during sets in shaded areas.* ***NOTE: Perform Weight-plyo techniques*** *(Chapter 9)* **on first 3 to 5 reps per set.**						
Chest	Bench press 2/12 Incline press 1/12 Chest stretch 30 sec	_____ _____		▓		▓		▓	
Back	Pull downs 2/12 Up back stretch 30 sec	_____		▓		▓		▓	
Shoulders	Shoulder press 2/10 Bent laterals 1/10 Shrugs 1/20 Shoulder stretch 30 sec Rotator cuff 1/15	_____ _____ _____ _____		▓		▓		▓	
Biceps	Curls 2/10 Incl DB curls 1/10	_____ _____		▓		▓		▓	
Triceps	Press downs 3/20	_____		▓		▓		▓	
Quads	Leg press 2/20 Leg ext 1/20	_____		▓		▓		▓	
Hamstrings	Leg curls 1/15 Stiff leg dead lift 1/10	_____		▓		▓		▓	
Calves	3-way calf raises 1/21	_____		▓		▓		▓	
Abs	Leg raises 1/20 Crunches 1/25	_____		▓		▓		▓	
Obliques	Twists 1/20	_____		▓		▓		▓	

STRATEGIC FITNESS PLAN

Training Log   Level Two   Week 4   Date_____

Workout:	Training Plan:		M	T	W	Th	F	Sat	S
10-Minute Stretching	**3 x week (M, Th, F)** *Chapter 6*		▩			▩	▩		
Cardio *Chapter 7*	**30 minutes 1 x week** *Tuesday or Thursday*			▩					
Sprint 8 *Chapter 8*	**20 minutes 2 x week** *30-50% speed/intensity during first 4 weeks. 8 reps 70 yards.*		▩			▩			
Plyometrics *Chapter 9*	**15 minutes 1 x week** *1 set plyo-drills*						▩		
Weight Training:	**Exercise:** *Chapter 10*	**Record Sets & Reps Performance** *sets/reps*		*Record amount of weight used during sets in shaded areas.* ***NOTE: Perform Weight-plyo techniques*** *(Chapter 9)* ***on first 3 to 5 reps per set.***					
Chest	Bench press 2/12	_____	▩	▩	▩	▩	▩	▩	
	Chest flys 1/12	_____							
	Chest stretch 30 sec								
Back	Pull downs 2/12	_____	▩	▩	▩	▩	▩	▩	
	Up back stretch 30 sec								
Shoulders	Shoulder press 2/10	_____	▩	▩	▩	▩	▩	▩	
	Side laterals 1/10	_____							
	Shrugs 1/20	_____							
	Shoulder stretch 30 sec								
Biceps	Curls 2/10	_____	▩	▩	▩	▩	▩	▩	
	Hammer curls 1/10								
Triceps	Press downs 2/20	_____	▩	▩	▩	▩	▩	▩	
	Triceps ext 1/12								
Quads	Hack squats 2/20	_____	▩	▩	▩	▩	▩	▩	
	Leg ext 1/20								
Hamstrings	Leg curls 1/15		▩	▩	▩	▩	▩	▩	
Calves	3-way calf raises 1/21	_____	▩	▩	▩	▩	▩	▩	
	Rev calf raises 1/20								
Abs	Crunches 2/25		▩	▩	▩	▩	▩	▩	
Obliques	Side bends 1/20								

NOTES:

NOTE: Continue the Fitness Plan for this Level until you complete your initial Eight-Week Commitment. For program continuation, additional copies of the Strategic Fitness Plans may be obtained from www.readysetgofitness.com. All purchasers of this book have permission to copy plans for personal use. After the initial eight weeks of training, repeat the Fitness Level adding intensity (more weight, reps, speed), or move to the next Fitness Level.

STRATEGIC FITNESS PLAN

Exercise Prescription - Level Three

MONDAY	TUESDAY	WEDNESDAY	THURSDAY	FRIDAY	SATURDAY	SUNDAY
10-Minute Stretching Routine *Chapter 6*	**Weights** 1 hour *Chapter 10*	**10-Minute Stretching Routine**	**10-Minute Stretching Routine**	**10-Minute Stretching Routine**	**Weights** 1 hour	Rest
Sprint 8 20 minutes *Chapter 8*	**Cardio-20** 20 minutes *Chapter 7*	*Make up day*	**Weights** 1 hour	**Sprint 8**	**Plyometrics** *Chapter 9*	
						TOTAL WEEK TIME:
30 minutes	1 hour 20 minutes	10 minutes	1 hour 10 minutes	30 minutes	1 hour 20 minutes	5 hours

STRATEGIC FITNESS PLAN

Training Log   Level Three   Week 1   Date_____

Workout:	Training Plan:		M	T	W	Th	F	Sat	S
10-Minute Stretching	**4 x week (M, W, Th, F)** *Chapter 6*		▒		▒	▒	▒		
Cardio *Chapter 7*	**30 minutes 1 x week** *Tuesday or Thursday*			▒					
Sprint 8 *Chapter 8*	**20 minutes 2 x week** *90-95% speed/intensity. 8 reps 70-yards*		▒		▒				
Plyometrics *Chapter 9*	**20 minutes 1 x week** *1 set plyo-drills*						▒		

Weight Training:	Exercise: *Chapter 10*		Record Sets & Reps Performance *sets/reps*	Record amount of weight used during sets in shaded areas. **NOTE: Perform weight-plyo techniques** (Chapter 9) **on first 3 to 5 reps per set.**					

Muscle	Exercise	sets/reps	Performance	M	T	W	Th	F	Sat	S
Chest	Bench press	3/12		▒						
	Incline press	2/12		▒						
	Cable flys	1/10		▒						
	Chest stretch	30 sec		▒						
	Pullovers	1/20		▒						
Back	Pull downs	3/12			▒					
	Cable rows	1/12			▒					
	Up back stretch	30 sec			▒					
	Hyper ext	1/20			▒					
Shoulders	Shoulder press	3/10					▒			
	Front laterals	2/10					▒			
	Shrugs	2/20					▒			
	Shoulder stretch	30 sec					▒			
	Rotator cuff	1/15					▒			
Biceps	Curls	3/10					▒			
	Incl DB curls	2/10					▒			
Triceps	Press downs	3/20					▒			
	Kick backs	1/20					▒			
Quads	Leg press	3/20							▒	
	Leg ext	2/20							▒	
	Lunges	1/10							▒	
Hamstrings	Leg curls	2/20							▒	
Calves	3-way calf raises	3/30							▒	
	Rev calf raises	1/40							▒	
Abs	Leg raises	2/20		▒		▒		▒	▒	
	Crunches	1/25		▒		▒		▒	▒	
Obliques	Twists	1/20		▒		▒		▒	▒	

STRATEGIC FITNESS PLAN

Training Log Level Three Week 2 Date_____

Workout:	Training Plan:	M	T	W	Th	F	Sat	S
10-Minute Stretching	**4 x week (M, W, Th, F)** *Chapter 6*	▓		▓	▓	▓		
Cardio *Chapter 7*	**30 minutes 1 x week** *Tuesday or Thursday*		▓					
Sprint 8 *Chapter 8*	**20 minutes 2 x week** *90-95% speed/intensity. 8 reps 70-yards*	▓					▓	
Plyometrics *Chapter 9*	**20 minutes 1 x week** *1 set plyo-drills*						▓	

Weight Training:	Exercise: *Chapter 10*	Record Sets & Reps Performance *sets/reps*						

Record amount of weight used during sets in shaded areas. **NOTE: Perform weight-plyo techniques (Chapter 9) on first 3 to 5 reps per set.**

Weight Training:	Exercise:	Record Sets & Reps	M	T	W	Th	F	Sat	S
Chest	Bench press 3/12 Decline press 2/12 Cable flys 1/10 Chest stretch 30 sec Pullovers 1/20	▓		▓					
Back	Pull downs 3/12 Cable rows 1/12 Up back stretch 30 sec Hyper ext 1/20	▓		▓					
Shoulders	Shoulder press 3/10 Side laterals 2/10 Shrugs 2/20 Shoulder stretch 30 sec Rotator cuff 1/15	▓				▓			
Biceps	Curls 3/10 Bicep 21s 1/10	▓				▓			
Triceps	Press downs 3/20 French press 1/20	▓				▓			
Quads	Leg press 3/20 One leg ext 2/20	▓						▓	
Hamstrings	Leg curls 2/20 Stiff dead lift 1/10	▓						▓	
Calves	3-way calf raises 3/30	▓							
Abs	Leg raises 2/20 Crunches 1/25	▓		▓	▓	▓			
Obliques	Side bends 1/20	▓			▓		▓		

STRATEGIC FITNESS PLAN

Training Log   Level Three   Week 3   Date_____

Workout:	Training Plan:		M	T	W	Th	F	Sat	S
10-Minute Stretching	**4 x week (M, W, Th, F)** *Chapter 6*								
Cardio *Chapter 7*	**30 minutes 1 x week** *Tuesday or Thursday*								
Sprint 8 *Chapter 8*	**20 minutes 2 x week** *90-95% speed/intensity. 8 reps 70-yards*								
Plyometrics *Chapter 9*	**20 minutes 1 x week** *1 set plyo-drills*								
Weight Training:	**Exercise:** *Chapter 10*	**Record Sets & Reps Performance** *sets/reps*	*Record amount of weight used during sets in shaded areas.* **NOTE: Perform weight-plyo techniques** *(Chapter 9)* **on first 3 to 5 reps per set.**						
Chest	Bench press 3/12 Incline press 2/12 Cable flys 1/10 Chest stretch 30 sec Pullovers 1/20								
Back	Pull downs 3/12 T-bar rows 1/12 Up back stretch 30 sec Hyper ext 1/20								
Shoulders	Shoulder press 3/10 Front laterals 2/10 Shrugs 2/20 Shoulder stretch 30 sec Rotator cuff 1/15								
Biceps	Curls 3/10 Incl DB curls 2/10 Hammer curls 1/10								
Triceps	Press downs 3/20 Rev press downs 1/20								
Quads	Leg press 3/20 Leg ext 2/20 Lunges 1/10								
Hamstrings	Leg curls 2/20								
Calves	3-way calf raises 3/30 Rev calf raises 1/40								
Abs	Leg raises 2/20 Crunches 1/25								
Obliques	Twists 1/20								

STRATEGIC FITNESS PLAN

Training Log **Level Three** **Week 4** **Date**_____

Workout:	Training Plan:		M	T	W	Th	F	Sat	S
10-Minute Stretching	**4 x week (M, W, Th, F)** *Chapter 6*		▓		▓	▓	▓		
Cardio *Chapter 7*	**30 minutes 1 x week** *Tuesday or Thursday*			▓					
Sprint 8 *Chapter 8*	**20 minutes 2 x week** *90-95% speed/intensity. 8 reps 70-yards*		▓						
Plyometrics *Chapter 9*	**20 minutes 1 x week** *1 set plyo-drills*							▓	

Weight Training:	**Exercise:** *Chapter 10*		**Record Sets & Reps Performance** *sets/reps*	*Record amount of weight used during sets in shaded areas.* **NOTE: Perform weight-plyo techniques** *(Chapter 9)* **on first 3 to 5 reps per set.**					
Chest	Bench press	3/12	____	▓	▓				
	Decline press	2/12	____						
	Cable flys	1/10	____						
	Chest stretch	30 sec	____						
	Pullovers	1/20	____						
Back	Pull downs	3/12	____	▓	▓				
	Cable rows	1/12	____						
	Up back stretch	30 sec	____						
	Hyper ext	1/20	____						
Shoulders	Shoulder press	3/10	____		▓	▓			
	Side laterals	2/10	____						
	Shrugs	2/20	____						
	Shoulder stretch	30 sec	____						
	Rotator cuff	1/15	____						
Biceps	Curls	3/10	____			▓			
	Bicep 21s	1/10	____						
Triceps	Press downs	3/20	____				▓		
	Tricep ext	1/20	____						
Quads	Leg press	3/20	____						▓
	One leg ext	2/10	____						
Hamstrings	Leg curls	2/20	____						▓
	Stiff dead lift	1/10	____						
Calves	3-way calf raises	3/30	____						▓
Abs	Leg raises	2/20	____		▓		▓		
	Crunches	1/25	____						
Obliques	Side bends	1/20	____						

NOTES:

STRATEGIC FITNESS PLAN

Exercise Prescription - Level Four

MONDAY	TUESDAY	WEDNESDAY	THURSDAY	FRIDAY	SATURDAY	SUNDAY
10-Minute Stretching Routine *Chapter 6*	**10-Minute Stretching Routine**		**10-Minute Stretching Routine**		**10-Minute Stretching Routine**	Rest
Sprint 8 20 minutes *Chapter 8*	**Plyometrics** 20 minutes *Chapter 9*	*Make up day*	**Sprint 8**	**Cardio-30** *Chapter 7*	**Sprint 8**	
Weights 1 hour *Chapter 10*	**Weights** 1 hour		**Weights** 1 hour		**Weights** 1 hour	
						TOTAL WEEK TIME:
1 hour 30 minutes	1 hour 30 minutes		1 hour 30 minutes	30 minutes	1 hour 30 minutes	6 hours 30 minutes

Before beginning Level Four, you should be experienced in sprinting, weightlifting, and the other components of Synergy Fitness.

STRATEGIC FITNESS PLAN

Training Log   Level Four   Week 1   Date_____

Workout:	Training Plan:		M	T	W	Th	F	Sat	S
10-Minute Stretching	**4 x week (M, T, Th, Sat)** *Chapter 6*								
Cardio *Chapter 7*	**30 minutes 1 x week** *Wednesday or Friday*								
Sprint 8 *Chapter 8*	**30 minutes 3 x week** *90-95% speed/intensity. 8 reps 70-yards*								
Plyometrics *Chapter 9*	**20 minutes 1 x week** *Tuesday or Saturday*								
Weight Training:	**Exercise:** *Chapter 10*	**Record Sets & Reps Performance** *sets/reps*	*Record amount of weight used during sets in shaded areas.* ***NOTE: Perform weight-plyo techniques*** *(Chapter 9)* ***on first 3 to 5 reps per set.***						
Chest	Bench press 3/12 Incline press 3/12 Cable flys 3/10 Chest stretch 30 sec								
Back	Pull downs 3/12 T-bar rows 3/12 Up back stretch 30 sec Hyper ext 1/20								
Shoulders	Shoulder press 3/10 Front laterals 3/10 Shrugs 3/20 Shoulder stretch 30 sec Rotator cuff 1/15								
Biceps	Curls 3/10 Incl DB curls 3/10								
Triceps	Press downs 3/20 Kick backs 2/20								
Quads	Leg press 3/20 Leg ext 3/20 Lunges 3/10								
Hamstrings	Leg curls 3/20								
Calves	3-way calf raises 3/20 Rev calf raises 1/40								
Abs	Leg raises 3/20 Crunches 2/25								
Obliques	Twists 1/30								

STRATEGIC FITNESS PLAN

Training Log   Level Four   Week 2   Date_____

Workout:	Training Plan:	M	T	W	Th	F	Sat	S
10-Minute Stretching	**4 x week (M, T, Th, Sat)** *Chapter 6*	▓	▓		▓		▓	
Cardio *Chapter 7*	**30 minutes 1 x week** *Wednesday or Friday*					▓		
Sprint 8 *Chapter 8*	**30 minutes 3 x week** *90-95% speed/intensity. 8 reps 70-yards*	▓		▓		▓		
Plyometrics *Chapter 9*	**20 minutes 1 x week** *Tuesday or Saturday*		▓					

Weight Training:	Exercise: *Chapter 10*	Record Sets & Reps Performance *sets/reps*	Record amount of weight used during sets in shaded areas. ***NOTE: Perform weight-plyo techniques (Chapter 9) on first 3 to 5 reps per set.***					
Chest	Bench press 3/12 Decline press 3/12 Chest flys 3/10 Chest stretch 30 sec	▓	▓			▓		
Back	Pull downs 3/12 Cable rows 3/12 Up back stretch 30 sec Hyper ext 1/20	▓			▓			
Shoulders	Shoulder press 3/10 Side laterals 3/10 Shrugs 3/20 Shoulder stretch 30 sec Rotator cuff 2/12	▓			▓			
Biceps	Curls 3/10 Incl DB curls 3/10 Forearm curls 2/10	▓					▓	
Triceps	Press downs 3/20 French press 2/20	▓					▓	
Quads	Leg press 3/20 Front squats 2/20 Leg ext 3/10	▓	▓					
Hamstrings	Leg curls 3/20	▓	▓					
Calves	3-way calf raises 3/20	▓	▓					
Abs	Leg raises 3/20 Crunches 2/25	▓	▓		▓		▓	
Obliques	Side bends 1/30	▓	▓		▓		▓	

STRATEGIC FITNESS PLAN

Training Log **Level Four** **Week 3** **Date**_____

Workout:	Training Plan:	M	T	W	Th	F	Sat	S
10-Minute Stretching	**4 x week (M, T, Th, Sat)** *Chapter 6*							
Cardio *Chapter 7*	**30 minutes 1 x week** *Wednesday or Friday*							
Sprint 8 *Chapter 8*	**30 minutes 3 x week** *90-95% speed/intensity. 8 reps 70-yards*							
Plyometrics *Chapter 9*	**20 minutes 1 x week** *Tuesday or Saturday*							

Weight Training:	Exercise: *Chapter 10*	Record Sets & Reps Performance *sets/reps*	Record amount of weight used during sets in shaded areas. **NOTE: Perform weight-plyo techniques (Chapter 9) on first 3 to 5 reps per set.**				
Chest	Bench press 3/12 Incline press 3/12 Chest flys 3/10 Pullovers 1/25 Chest stretch 30 sec						
Back	Pull downs 3/12 T-bar rows 3/12 Up back stretch 30 sec Hyper ext 1/20						
Shoulders	Shoulder press 3/10 Front laterals 3/10 Bent laterals 1/15 Shrugs 3/20 Shoulder stretch 30 sec Rotator cuff 2/15						
Biceps	Curls 3/10 Incl DB curls 3/10 Bicep 21s 1 set						
Triceps	Press downs 3/20 Tricep ext 3/20						
Quads	Squats 3/10 Leg ext 3/20 Hip Flex 2/10						
Hamstrings	Leg curls 3/20 Stiff dead lift 1/10						
Calves	3-way calf raises 3/20						
Abs	Leg raises 3/20 Crunches 2/25						
Obliques	Twists 1/30						

STRATEGIC FITNESS PLAN

Training Log   Level Four   Week 4   Date_____

Workout:	Training Plan:		M	T	W	Th	F	Sat	S
10-Minute Stretching	**4 x week (M, T, Th, Sat)** *Chapter 6*		▓	▓		▓		▓	
Cardio *Chapter 7*	**30 minutes 1 x week** *Wednesday or Friday*						▓		
Sprint 8 *Chapter 8*	**30 minutes 3 x week** *90-95% speed/intensity. 8 reps 70-yards*		▓		▓		▓		
Plyometrics *Chapter 9*	**20 minutes 1 x week** *Tuesday or Saturday*			▓					

Weight Training:	Exercise: *Chapter 10*	Record Sets & Reps Performance *sets/reps*	M	T	W	Th	F	Sat	S
		Record amount of weight used during sets in shaded areas. **NOTE: Perform weight-plyo techniques (Chapter 9) on first 3 to 5 reps per set.**							
Chest	Bench press 3/12 Incline press 3/12 Dips 3/10 Pullovers 1/25 Chest stretch 30 sec		▓						
Back	Pull downs 3/12 Cable rows 3/12 Up back stretch 30 sec Hyper ext 1/20					▓			
Shoulders	Sh press 3/10 Side laterals 3/10 Bent laterals 3/10 Shrugs 3/20 Shoulder stretch 30 sec Rotator cuff 2/15								
Biceps	Curls 3/10 Incl DB curls 3/10 Bicep 21s 1 set Hammer curls 2/12							▓	
Triceps	Press downs 3/20 Tricep ext 2/15 Rev French press 1/15							▓	
Quads	Leg press 3/20 Hack squats 2/15 One leg L. ext 3/20 Lunges 2/10			▓					
Hamstrings	Leg curls 3/20			▓					
Calves	3-way calf raises 3/20 Rev calf raises 1/40			▓					
Abs	Leg raises 3/20 Crunches 2/25					▓		▓	
Obliques	Side bends 1/30					▓		▓	

NOTES:

NOTE: Continue the Fitness Plan for this Level until you complete your initial Eight-Week Commitment. For program continuation, additional copies of the Strategic Fitness Plans may be obtained from www.readysetgofitness.com. All purchasers of this book have permission to copy plans for personal use. After the initial eight-weeks of training, repeat the Fitness Level adding intensity (more weight, reps, speed), or move to the next Fitness Level.

STRATEGIC FITNESS PLAN

Exercise Prescription - Level Five

MONDAY	TUESDAY	WEDNESDAY	THURSDAY	FRIDAY	SATURDAY	SUNDAY
10-Minute Stretching Routine *Chapter 6*	**10-Minute Stretching Routine**		**10-Minute Stretching Routine**	**10-Minute Stretching Routine**	**10-Minute Stretching Routine**	Rest
Sprints *Chapter 8*	**Plyometrics** 20 minutes *Chapter 9*	*Make up day*	**Plyometrics** 20 minutes	**Cardio-30** *Chapter 7*	**Sprints:** 8x100 meters 8x20 Bleacher runs 10 sets (walk down bleachers)	
Program A: 8x60 meters 4x150 meters						
Alternate with ***Program B:*** 4 sets of: 1x60 meters 1x150 1x300	**Sprints:** 10x40 meters 10x20		**Sprints:** Sprint ladder: 2x60 meters 2x100 2x200 2x100 2x60			
*1 minute rest between sprints. *2 minutes rest between sets.						
Weights 1 hour *Chapter 10*	**Weights** 1 hour		**Weights** 1 hour	**Weights** 1 hour	**Weights** 1 hour	
2 hour s 30 minutes	2 hours		2 hours 30 minutes	1 hour 30 minutes	2 hours 30 minutes	**TOTAL WEEK TIME:** 12 hours

Level Five is the maximum program designed for off season college and professional athletes. It is set up to be a four-week rotation. Heavy Olympic and power lifting are prescribed for one day a week (Saturdays). The weight training routine is set for five days in the gym. Should you encounter time problems, the following split-routine could be substituted for a four-day-week split: Day 1, chest/back; Day 2, legs; Day 3, shoulders/arms; Day 4, plyo-lifts.

Plyo-power Lifting
One day a week, four-week rotation

Week 1 Training Plan *(Sat)*	Performance *Weight sets / reps*
Power Cleans 3 x 3-5	lbs
Squats 5 x 3-5	lbs

Week 2 Training Plan	Performance *Weight sets / reps*
Push presses 3 x 8-12	lbs
Dead lifts 3 x 3-5	lbs

Week 3 Training Plan	Performance *Weight sets / reps*
Power Cleans 3 x 3-5	lbs
One leg squats 3 x 10	lbs

Week 4 Training Plan	Performance *Weight sets / reps*
Push presses 3 x 8-12	lbs
Squats 3 x 8	lbs

Strategic Fitness Plan Level Five is demanding. No, it's very demanding. But it will produce great results! The goal is high-intensity **injury-free training**. Listen to your body. Injury-free training during the off-season is important in maximizing results. And Remember the Isshinryu 90 percent extension rule covered in Chapter 9.

STRATEGIC FITNESS PLAN

Training Log   **Level Five**   **Week 1**   **Date_____**

Workout:	Training Plan:		M	T	W	Th	F	Sat	S
10-Minute Stretching	**4 x week (M, T, Th, Sat)** *Chapter 6*								
Cardio *Chapter 7*	**30 minutes 2 x week** *Cardio is also multi-tasked with anaerobic training*								
Sprint 8 *Chapter 8*	**30 minutes 3 x week** *90-95% speed/intensity. See Exercise Prescription.*								
Plyometrics *Chapter 9*	**20 minutes 2 x week** *2 sets plyo-drills*								

Weight Training:	Exercise: *Chapter 10*	Record Sets & Reps Performance *sets/reps*	Record amount of weight used during sets in shaded areas. **NOTE: Perform weight-plyo techniques (Chapter 9) on first 3 to 5 reps per set.**						
Chest	Bench press 3/8 Incline press 3/12 Dips 3/10 Cable flys 3/10 Chest stretch 30 sec							Plyo-power lifts on Saturday	
Back	Pull downs 5/12 Dumbbell rows 3/12 Up back stretch 30 sec Hyper ext 2/15								
Shoulders	Sh press 5/8 Front laterals 3/10 Bent laterals 3/10 Shrugs 3/20 Shoulder stretch 30 sec Rotator cuff 2/15								
Biceps	Curls 5/10 Incl DB curls 3/10 Bicep 21s 3 sets Forearm curls 2/10								
Triceps	Press downs 3/20 Kick backs 3/20 Rev press downs 3/15								
Quads	Leg press 3/20 One leg squats 3/10 Leg ext 3/20 Lunges 3/10								
Hamstrings	Leg curls 3/20 Stiff leg dead lift 1/10								
Calves	3-way calf raises 3/20 Rev calf raises 1/50								
Abs	Leg raises 3/20 Crunches 2/20								
Obliques	Side bends 1/30								

STRATEGIC FITNESS PLAN

Training Log **Level Five** **Week 2** **Date**_____

Workout:	Training Plan:		M	Tu	W	Th	F	Sat	S
10-Minute Stretching	**4 x week (M, T, Th, Sat)** *Chapter 6*		▓	▓		▓		▓	
Cardio *Chapter 7*	**30 minutes 2 x week**		▓		▓		▓		
Sprint 8 *Chapter 8*	**30 minutes 3 x week** *90-95% speed/intensity*		▓		▓		▓	▓	
Plyometrics *Chapter 9*	**20 minutes 2 x week** *2 sets plyo-drills*		▓		▓				

Weight Training:	Exercise: *Chapter 10*		**Record Sets & Reps Performance** *sets/reps*		*Record amount of weight used during sets in shaded areas.* ***NOTE: Perform weight-plyo techniques** (Chapter 9) **on first 3 to 5 reps per set.***

Chest	Bench press	3/8	▓		
	Incline press	3/12			
	Decline press	3/10			
	D/B flys	3/10			
	Pullovers	1/25			
	Chest stretch	30 sec			

Plyo-power lifts on Saturday

Section	Exercises	M	Tu	W	Th	F	Sat	S
Back	Pull downs 5/12 / Cable rows 3/12 / Up back stretch 30 sec / Hyper ext 2/20	▓			▓			
Shoulders	Sh press 5/8 / Side laterals 3/10 / Bent laterals 3/10 / Shrugs 3/20 / Shoulder stretch 30 sec / Rotator cuff 2/15	▓			▓			
Biceps	Curls 5/10 / Incl DB curls 3/10 / Bicep 21s 3 sets / Hammer curls 2/10	▓					▓	
Triceps	Press downs 3/20 / Tricep ext 3/20 / Kick backs 3/15	▓						
Quads	Leg press 3/20 / Hack squats 3/10 / Leg ext 3/20 / Hip flexors Rev 2/10	▓						
Hamstrings	Leg curls 5/20	▓						
Calves	3-way calf raises 6/20	▓						
Abs	Leg raises 3/25 / Crunches 2/30	▓						
Obliques	Twists 1/30	▓						

STRATEGIC FITNESS PLAN

Training Log   Level Five   Week 3   Date_____

Workout:	Training Plan:		M	T	W	Th	F	Sat	S
10-Minute Stretching	**4 x week (M, T, Th, Sat)** *Chapter 6*		▓	▓		▓		▓	
Cardio *Chapter 7*	**30 minutes 2 x week**				▓		▓		
Sprint 8 *Chapter 8*	**30 minutes 3 x week** *90-95% speed/intensity*		▓		▓		▓		
Plyometrics *Chapter 9*	**20 minutes 2 x week** *2 sets plyo-drills*		▓			▓			
Weight Training:	**Exercise:** *Chapter 10*	**Record Sets & Reps Performance** *sets/rreps*	*Record amount of weight used during sets in shaded areas.* **NOTE: Perform weight-plyo techniques (Chapter 9) on first 3 to 5 reps per set.**						
Chest	Bench press 3/8 / Incline press 3/12 / Dips 3/10 / Cable flys 3/10 / Chest stretch 30 sec	▓	▓					Plyo-power lifts on Saturday	
Back	Pull downs 5/12 / Cable rows 3/12 / Up back stretch 30 sec / Hyper ext 2/20	▓				▓			
Shoulders	Sh press 5/8 / Front laterals 3/10 / Bent laterals 3/10 / Shrugs 3/20 / Shoulder stretch 30 sec / Rotator cuff 2/15	▓				▓			
Biceps	Curls 5/10 / Incl DB curls 3/10 / Bicep 21s 3 sets / Forearm curls 2/10	▓					▓		
Triceps	Press downs 3/20 / French press 3/20 / Rev press downs 1/15	▓					▓		
Quads	Leg press 3/20 / One leg squats 3/10 / Leg ext 3/20 / Hip flexors 3/10	▓		▓					
Hamstrings	Leg curls 3/20 / Stiff leg dead lift 1/10	▓		▓					
Calves	3-way calf raises 3/20 / Rev calf raises 1/50	▓		▓					
Abs	Leg raises 3/25 / Crunches 2/30	▓				▓	▓	▓	
Obliques	Side bends 1/30	▓							

STRATEGIC FITNESS PLAN

Training Log   **Level Five**   **Week 4**   **Date**_____

Workout:	Training Plan:	M	Tu	W	Th	F	Sat	S
10-Minute Stretching	**4 x week (M, T, Th, Sat)** *Chapter 6*	▓	▓		▓		▓	
Cardio *Chapter 7*	**30 minutes 2 x week**			▓			▓	
Sprint 8 *Chapter 8*	**30 minutes 3 x week** *90-95% speed/intensity*	▓		▓		▓		
Plyometrics *Chapter 9*	**20 minutes 2 x week** *2 sets plyo-drills*		▓		▓			

Weight Training:	Exercise: *Chapter 10*	Record Sets & Reps Performance *sets/rreps*	Record amount of weight used during sets in shaded areas. **NOTE: Perform weight-plyo techniques (Chapter 9) on first 3 to 5 reps per set.**					
Chest	Bench press 3/8 Incline press 3/12 Decline press 3/10 Cable flys 3/10 Pullovers 1/25 Chest stretch 30 sec						Plyo-power lifts on Saturday	
Back	Pull downs 5/12 T-bar rows 3/12 Up back stretch 30 sec Hyper ext 2/20							
Shoulders	Sh press 5/8 Side laterals 3/10 Bent laterals 3/10 Shrugs 3/20 Shoulder stretch 30 sec Rotator cuff 2/15							
Biceps	Curls 5/10 Incl DB curls 3/10 Bicep 21s 3 sets Hammer curls 2/10							
Triceps	Press downs 3/20 French press 3/20 Rev press downs 3/15							
Quads	Leg press 3/20 Front squats 3/10 Leg ext -one leg 3/20 Lunges 2/10							
Hamstrings	Leg curls 5/20							
Calves	3-way calf raises 6/20							
Abs	Leg raises 3/25 Crunches 2/30							
Obliques	Twists 1/30							

Conclusion

The single most important aspect of health and fitness improvement is discussed in this conclusion. This one aspect cannot be sold in a nutrition store, obtained with a physician's prescription pad, or purchased at a gym. The single most important aspect of fitness improvement is absolutely free.

This issue is so fundamental that even with the medical research information from this book and a Strategic Fitness Plan as a guide, this one aspect will ultimately determine the success of your fitness program.

If not accomplished, this one issue stands in the way of achieving a new appearance, feeling great about yourself, and raising your health and fitness to new levels. The most important fitness component is the commitment you make to follow a Strategic Fitness Plan for the first eight weeks.

In the first eight weeks, you need 100 percent determination to stay with your Strategic Fitness Plan.

While this book was written to be a life long exercise prescription, we need short-range goals to determine if we are on the correct course toward long-range objectives. The first eight weeks are critically important and will make or break your fitness improvement effort.

> **Researchers demonstrate that signing a statement of commitment expressing intent to train will significantly increase success.** *(Facilitating changes in exercise behavior: effect of structured statements of intention on perceived barriers to action,* 1995, Huddy).

There are several factors that might keep you from making a serious commitment to begin and stick with a total fitness program: perceived barriers, past experience, or fear of failure or embarrassment, (*Use of attitude-behavior models in exercise promotion,* 1990, Godin).

These are natural human emotions that need to be worked through. The best way to do this is simply to understand that these are natural feelings felt by everyone beginning a new program, and press on.

A research test group that had signed a structured "statement of intent for an exercise plan" that addressed major barriers" had a twofold increase in frequency and intensity of exercise over the control group that did not sign the statement.

At the end of the following discussion concerning what happens during the first eight weeks of training, there is a commitment form you should seriously consider signing. This will formalize your eight-week commitment—to you!

Major barriers that might deter you from achieving your eight-week commitment should be thought through. And action plans to overcome each barrier should be developed before signing. These barriers might be work schedule, family responsibility, travel schedule, and gym or home equipment availability. You should develop a specific action plan to deal with each one.

SYNERGY FITNESS STRATEGY 10
Make the Eight-Week Commitment

The First Eight Weeks

Physiologists tell us, when starting something new (like the Strategic Fitness Plan), we are enthusiastic initially and go through four phases before the new activity becomes internalized and becomes part of us. The four phases are: *Form, Storm, Norm,* and *Perform.*

The *Form* phase is marked with the excitement of beginning a new program. During the first week of your fitness plan, sticking with the plan should be easy. You may even feel you can handle more training. Don't do this. Not only does overtraining risk injury, it risks your motivation and continuation of the fitness program over time.

One main mental deterrent occurs in this phase— waiting for all the lights to turn green before beginning. While preparation is good, pick a start date. Go for it. And don't look back.

The *Storm* phase follows a few weeks later. When we learn the program is hard work (on some days), and we just don't want to train—this is the storm phase. And it happens to everyone.

In the *Storm* phase, we begin to create excuses (conscious and subconscious) for missing workouts. This is by far the toughest phase.

How should you get through this phase? Mentally prepare ahead of time. The *Storm* phase is a natural phase that everyone experiences. The key to overcoming it is to make the commitment now to press through the *Storm* phase when it occurs. And it will occur. Don't let this natural human emotion deter you from your fitness goal.

Consistency is a must during the initial eight weeks. Following your Strategic Fitness Plan will improve appearance and produce fitness gains rapidly. The positive results will increase satisfaction, motivation, and, subsequently, improve the results of training.

Research from Stamford University demonstrates that dieters who were dissatisfied with their bodies only have a 36 percent success rate with a diet and exercise program. Dieters more satisfied with their bodies have a 63 percent success rate. (Characteristics of successful and unsuccessful dieters: an application of signal detection methodology, 1998, Kiernan).

The *Norm* phase is adapting to your fitness training commitment by learning that you can press through the tough days when you do not feel like training and still get in a great workout. Every successful, long-term training individual knows—feeling bad at the beginning of the workout, often means this will be the best workout of the week.

The *Perform* phase occurs when you have experienced the first three phases and begin to train consistently. It is when fitness training becomes internalized.

Repetition eventually becomes habit, and that is the goal of this fitness program. Training can't be a choice. Fitness training is just something that you do. It must become a part of who you are. This is the *Perform* phase.

During the first eight weeks, you will not only be making positive physical changes, but there will be positive mental changes as well. Don't make the mistake of thinking that you will bypass the first three phases and go straight to the *Perform* phase. This is a mistake. When this happens, the *Storm* phase seems to forcefully pop up and pull the person back into this phase.

A better strategy is to simply be mentally prepared for all four phases in advance. Identify the phase you are experiencing, and with maturity and confidence, work through the mental aspects of training by sticking to the plan on the tough days.

When you reach the *Perform* phase, maintaining the fitness plan is much easier. But you can't get there until the first eight weeks are completed. Completing the Fitness Success Plan work sheet (right) will be helpful.

Fitness Success Plan

Barriers to the success of following your Strategic Fitness Plan for eight weeks:

Action plans to overcome barriers:

It is time to make the Eight Week Commitment. This is a formal promise . . . to you . . . that you will follow your Strategic Fitness Plan consistently for eight weeks.

The Eight-Week Commitment

I _____ commit on this day_____
     (Print your name)   (Today's date)

to carefully select the appropriate Fitness Level based on

age, training experience, and fitness level: _____
                        (Select Fitness Level One through Five)

and will follow the Strategic Fitness Plan for eight-weeks.

_____
             (Sign)

Date: Mission Accomplished_____
Return to this page after completing the eight-weeks of fitness training and in big print write the date you accomplished this important goal. Then review the section "Long-Term Fitness Training."

Long-Term Fitness Training

The key to long-term training is to be aware that motivation comes and goes, and comes and goes. The one day that you decide to miss could be the last workout for a year. Long-term training is not a physical issue, it is a mental one.

I have a mental practice that I use to help me through the tough days when I do not feel like training. I do not make the decision to miss a workout until I first change into my training clothes. If I decide to miss a workout, that is okay (sometimes it's unavoidable), but I always make the effort to change clothes first.

Most of the time, just changing into training clothes is enough to get me started training. Once started, this typically becomes the best workout of the week.

Everyone who has stopped exercising began by "missing once." That one miss led to another, then another. The key to long-term training is to understand the mental risk associated with missing "one workout."

I cannot overemphasize the importance of mentally making an issue of missing "one workout." Missing a workout will not hurt you physically. Mentally, however, missing a workout permanently breaks the habit of training—until you make the next workout. When deciding to miss, tell yourself that you just decided to "permanently stop training" until you have completed the next workout.

Researchers show that lifelong exercise can counteract the effects associated with aging of the neuromuscular system. (Effects of strength and endurance training on skeletal muscles in the elderly. New muscles for old! 1999, Lexell).

Ten Synergy Fitness Strategies

The health and fitness information presented in this book is reliable. It is supported by medical research and will produce positive results rapidly.

Whether you are a physician writing an "exercise prescription" for patients, a marathoner looking to reduce time per mile and build strength in key areas for injury prevention, an athlete training for the upcoming season, a bodybuilder seeking to improve symmetry by reducing percentage of body fat while adding lean muscle, a patient with joint disease following physicians orders, or middle-aged and wanting to get into shape, following one of the five Strategic Fitness Plans in the preceding chapter will help you achieve your goals.

Reading this book, you have learned Ten Fitness Strategies that are worth reviewing periodically.

Ten Synergy Fitness Strategies

1. Increase growth hormone naturally

2. Reach GH release benchmarks during fitness training
    - Out-of-breath (oxygen debt)
    - Muscle burn (lactic acid)
    - Increased body temperature
    - Adrenal response (slightly painful)

3. Maximize GH release during fitness training
    Before training: No high fat meals one hour prior
    During training: Drink lots of water
    After training: No sugar for two hours
    Intake 25 grams of protein

4. Get adequate "slow wave" deep sleep

5. Maintain insulin balance through common-sense nutrition

6. Use GH-releasing exercise targeting the body's three energy systems

7. Use The Target Zone Training Method by targeting slow-twitch, and fast-twitch IIa & IIx muscle fiber during training

8. Use a comprehensive strategic fitness plan to increase flexibility, endurance, anaerobic capacity, strength, and power

9. During resistance training, isolate muscles being worked, train every set to exhaustion, aerobically

10. Make the Eight-Week Commitment

Concluding Thoughts

Current society dictates that Olympic athletes are thought to be over the hill at age 20 in some sports. It is rare to see a gymnast over age 25. This is because our view of competition is limited and narrow.

Our current definition of competition is based on the single limited absolute...winning. Do not misunderstand. I love competition. I think the national health problem in America is due to the lack of competition and a new definition of competition would begin to cure the current national health crisis.

We have the Senior Olympics and the Special Olympics. What we need is the Masters Olympics for age 30 and up (with incentives for as many participants as possible). Most people stop competing in physical events after high school. A small number continue in college through intramurals and official athletic competitions. And unless you are in that very small number making it to the pros, almost all competition is over—for life. This is a huge cultural failure.

This view of competition leaves us with essentially "slow-twitch" muscle developing competitions—with perhaps tennis and softball being the exceptions. The only widespread competitions available are marathons. However, the amount of training time required makes this event impractical for most people with active careers and children to raise.

Most are unaware of master's competitions in swimming, cycling, and track and field.

Competition is a healthy aspect of human nature when used constructively. Competition can be destructive. On the news, we see parents fill their missing need for competition by fighting and injuring others over their children's games. As a nation, we need to create healthy and meaningful competition for adults of all ages.

The physical benefits of maintaining competition throughout life would be enormous. In my humble opinion, this would cure the nation's health problem. Just as a physician writes an "exercise prescription," physicians (not physician organizations), but individual, actively practicing physicians, must accept the leadership role in curing the national health problem. Educators seeing obesity becoming an epidemic in schools, and health officials also have an important role.

We have health information everywhere. And it is not working. In fact, as more and more health information becomes available, Americans somehow become less and less healthy.

What we need is the *motivation* to get fit. And healthy competition for middle-aged and older adults could provide motivation for many. Rather than telling people to lose weight and exercise, perhaps encouragement to begin training for a 200-meter race for the next Senior Olympics competition, or masters event would provide motivation.

It was once thought that a selective loss of fast-twitch muscle fiber occurred naturally with aging. New research shows that this is not true. Fitness training—even at ages above 70 years, can develop fast-twitch muscle fiber that is necessary for anaerobic exercise.

"Decreased physical activity with aging appears to be the key factor involved in producing sarcopenia, *(loss of muscle and strength during aging)"* (Sarcopenia, 2001, Morley). Researchers show that the medical condition of muscles wasting (sarcopenia) is also implicated with the decrease of growth hormone during aging. And Sarcopenia occurs with a "disproportionate atrophy (wasting) of fast-twitch muscle fibers."

Researchers demonstrate that older men (age 52-62) experience a decrease of type II muscle fiber during aging; however, training can prevent this effect of aging, (Oxidative capacity of human muscle fiber types: effects of age and training status, 1995, Proctor).

In short, if we do not continue to train all three muscle fiber types during aging, we lose the ability to increase growth hormone because we no longer have fast-twitch muscle fiber that is necessary for anaerobic exercise.

Researchers at Ball State University prove that older men (average age 74) could increase muscle cell size, strength, velocity of movement, and power in both slow and fast-twitch muscle fiber, (*Effect of resistance training on single muscle fiber contractile function in older men*, 2000, Trappe).

This research also demonstrates that fast-twitch fiber is not activated until the exercise reaches a certain level of high-intensity effort. This fact serves as the basis for the need for widespread, competitions for adults that emphasize fast-twitch muscle development like masters track and field, swimming and cycling.

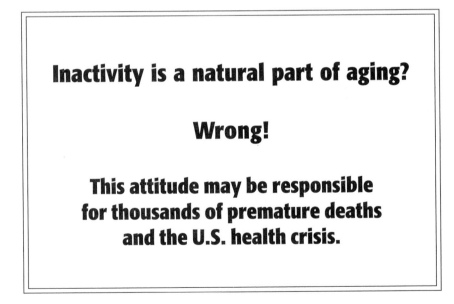

Inactivity is a natural part of aging?

Wrong!

This attitude may be responsible for thousands of premature deaths and the U.S. health crisis.

Healthy Competition

As we age, without healthy competition and anaerobic exercise programs to sustain the use of fast-twitch muscle fiber, our "society of convenience" motivates us to allow the fast-twitch fiber developed in youth to atrophy and simply waste away during aging.

We do not recognize the fast-twitch atrophy as it occurs, because most activity (after high school and college) is in slow-twitch mode.

Looking through a microscope at muscle cells during youth, you would see a uniformity of cells and the proper distribution of the three muscle fiber types—slow twitch, and fast twitch IIa, and the super fast IIx.

Looking at older muscles under a microscope, you would see some uniformity with the slow-twitch muscle cells along with an unorganized group of fast-twitch muscle cells that have atrophied and wasted away over time.

To maintain fitness for a lifetime, it is not sufficient to exercise in the traditional manner. Jogging will develop your slow-twitch muscle fiber in your legs. Bench press performed in the traditional "slow-squeeze-out-reps" mode will strengthen the slow-twitch fiber in your chest.

To achieve optimum fitness (and maintain it during aging), you will need to enter the new paradigm; a new way of thinking about health, fitness, and aging. The thinking needs to be focused on developing and maintaining all three muscle fiber types all major body parts—throughout life.

The Strategic Fitness Plan for your appropriate Fitness Level will accomplish *The Target Zone Method* of training and develop all three types of muscles in your body. Anaerobic sprint training, martial arts and some Olympic lifting, and plyometric drills will activate and develop the fast-twitch IIx fiber. Swimming, running intervals, biking, skiing—and plyo-weights will target the fast-twitch IIa fiber. And cardio and classical weight training will develop your slow-twitch muscle fiber.

The New Fitness Paradigm

Are we are entering a new paradigm of health and fitness? It is too early to tell. But there is hope.

Hot-off-the-press medical research certainly supports the need for a comprehensive fitness training model that includes (the missing ingredient) anaerobic training. The better question may be—how long will it take before physicians begin writing "exercise prescriptions" for their patients for comprehensive fitness training? Or, how long will it be before a major national focus is placed on reinventing healthy athletic competition for middle-aged adults that will target fast-twitch muscle fiber development?

There have been two major worldwide fitness revolutions—weightlifting in the 1960s and distance running in the 1980s

Famous U.S. weightlifting coach Bob Hoffman began promoting resistance training and endorsing weight training equipment in the 1960s. This movement caught fire and today in the United States there are 16,000 fitness centers and health clubs—up by 4,000 in recent years. Fitness centers are located in nearly every city across the country.

Many participated in the "endurance fitness" revolution in the 1980s. Dr. Kenneth Cooper wrote the book *Aerobics* and fired the starting gun for the world to begin jogging. We began believing that quantity and quality of life could be extended by jogging and performing aerobic exercise that achieved cardiac target rates 30 minutes a day.

Many benefited from the aerobics and weight training national movements. Cardiac fitness levels improved for its participants. However, it is time to implement new medical research and move to a comprehensive fitness model that includes high-intensity anaerobic training.

We have a national health fitness crisis in this country and I hope you will encourage family members, friends, and neighbors to join you and start a Synergy Fitness Group. Most of all, it is my hope you will implement the information presented in this book by making the Eight-Week Commitment, and improve your health, fitness, and appearance beyond your wildest imagination.

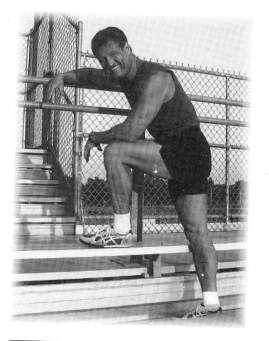

References

Introduction & Chapter 1

Atalay, Sen. (1999). "Physical exercise and antioxidant defenses in the heart." *Ann N Y Sci.* Jun30;874:169-77. PMID: 10415530.

Biolo, Maggi, Williams, Tipton, Wolfe. (1995). "Increased rates of muscle protein turnover and amino acid transport after resistance exercise in humans." *Am J Physiol.* Mar;268(3 Pt 1):E514-20. PMID: 7900797.

Cappon, Ipp, Brasel, Cooper. (1993). "Acute effects of high fats and high glucose meals on the growth hormone response to exercise." *J Clin Endocrinol Metab.* Jun;76(6):1418-22. PMID: 8501145.

Cheung, Zhao, Chait, Albers, Brown. (2001). "Antioxidant supplements block the response of hdl to simvastatin-niacin therapy in patients with coronary artery disease and low hdl." *Arterioscler Thromb Vasc Biol.* Aug;21(8):1320-6. PMID: 11498460.

Christensen, Jorgensen, Moller, Orskov. (1984). "Characterization of growth hormone release in response to external heating. Comparison to exercise induced release." *Acta Endocrinol.* Nov;107(3):295-301. PMID: 6507003.

Chwalbinski-Moneta. (1996). "Threshold increases in plasma growth hormone in relation to plasma catecholamine and blood lactate concentration during progressive exercise in endurance-trained athletes." *Eur J Appl Physiol Occup Physiol.* 73(1-2):117-20. PMID: 8861679.

Di Luigi, Guidetti, Nordio, Baldari, Romanelli. (2001). "Acute effect of physical Exercise on serum insulin-like growth factor-binding protein 2 and 3 in healthy men: role of exercise linked growth hormone secretion." *Int J Sports Med.* Feb;22(2):103-110. PMID: 11291611.

Di Luigi, Guidetti, Pigozzi, Baldari, Casini, Nordio, Romanelli. (1999). "Acute amino Acids supplementation enhances pituitary responsiveness in athletics." *Med Sci Sports Exerc.* Dec;31(12):1748-54. PMID: 10613424.

Eberhardt, Ingram, Makuc. (2001). Urban and Rural Health Chartbook. *Health, United States, 2001.* Hyattsville, Maryland: National Center for Health Statistics.

Elias, Wilson, Naqvi, Pandan. (1997). "Effects of blood pH and blood lactate on growth hormone, prolactin, and gonadotropin release after acute exercise in male volunteers. *Proc Soc Exp Biol Med.* Feb;214(2):156-60. PMID: 9034133.

Felsing, Brasel, Cooper. (1992). "Effect of low and high intensity exercise on circulating growth hormone in men. *J Clin Endocrinol Metab.* Jul;75(1):157-62. PMID: 1619005.

Frewin, Frantz, Downey. (1976). "The effect of ambient temperature on the growth hormone and prolactin response to exercise." *Aust J Exp Biol Med Sci.* Feb:54(1):97-101. PMID: 942365.

Groussard, Morel, Chevanne, Monnier, Cillard, Delamarche. (2000). Free radical scavenging and antioxidant effects of lactate ion: an in vitro study." *J Appl Physiol.* Jul;89(1):169-75. PMID: 10904049.

Kastello, Sothmann, Murthy. (1993). "Young and old subjects for aerobic capacity have similar noradrenergic responses to exercise." *J Appl Physiol.* Jan;74(1):49-54. PMID: 8444733.

Lemura, Von Duvillard, Mookerjee. (2000). "The effects of physical training on functional capacity in adults. Ages 46 to 90: a meta-analysis." *J Sports Med Phy Fitness.* Mar;40(1):1-10. PMID: 10822903.

Lugar. (1988). "Acute exercise stimulates the rennin-angiotensin-aldosterone axis adaptive changes in runners." *Horm Res.* 30(1);5-9. PMID: 2851526.

Meirleir, Naaktgeboren. (1986). "Beta-endorphin and ACTH levels in peripheral blood during and after aerobic and anaerobic exercise." *Eur J Appl Physiol Occup Physiol.* 55(1):5-8. PMID: 3009176.

MacIntyre, Reid, McKenzie. (1995). "Delayed muscle soreness. The inflammatory response to muscle injury and its clinical implications." *Sports Med.* Jul;20(1):24-40. PMID: 7481277.

Paw, De Jong, Pallast, Kloek, Schouten, Kok. (2000). "Immunity in frail elderly: a randomized controlled trial of exercise and enriched foods." *Med Sci Sports Exerc.* Dec:32(12):2005-11. PMID: 11128843.

Parise, Yarasheski. (2000). "The utility of resistance training and amino acid supplementation for reversing age-associated decrements in muscle protein mass and function." *Curr Opin Clin Nutr Metab Care.* Nov 3;(6):489-95. PMID:11085836.

Peyreigne, Bouix, Fedou, Mercier. (2001). "Effect of hydration on exercise-induced growth hormone." *Eur J Endocrinol.* Sept;145(4):445-50. PMID: 115810003.

Pritzlaff, Wideman, Weltman, J., Abbott, Gutgesell, Hartman, Veldhuis, Weltman, A. (2000). "Catecholamine release, growth hormone secretion, and energy expenditure during exercise vs. recovery in men." *J Appl Physiol.* Sept;89(3):937-46. PMID: 10956336.

Pritzlaff, Wideman, Weltman, J., Abbott, Gutgesell, Hartman, Veldhuis, Weltman, A. (2000). "Impact of acute exercise intensity on pulsatile growth hormone release in men." *J Appl Physiol.* Aug;87(2):498-504. PMID: 10444604.

Sutton, Lazarus. (1976). "Growth hormone in exercise: comparison of physiological and pharmacological stimuli." *J Appl Physiol.* Oct;41(4):523-7. PMID: 985395.

Terry, Willoughby, Braseau, Martin, Patel. (1976). "Antiserum to somatostatin prevents stress-induced inhibition of growth hormone secretion in the rat." *Science.* May 7;192(4239):565-7. PMID: 1257793.

Toogood, O'Neill, Shalet. (1996). "Beyond the somatopause: growth hormone deficiency in adults over the age of 60 years." *J Clin Endocrinol Metab.* Feb; 81(2):460-5. National Library of Science, PubMed abstract: 8636250.

Vanhelder, Radomski, Goode. (1984). "Growth hormone responses during intermittent weightlifting exercise in Men." *Eur J Physiol Occup Physiol.* 53(1):31-4. PMID: 6542499.

Vigas, Celko, Koska. (2000). "Role of body temperature in exercise-induced growth hormone and prolactin release in non-trained and physically fit subjects." Endocr Regul. Dec;34(4):175-180. PMID: 11137977.

Weltman, Weltman, Womack, Davis, Blumer, Gasser, Hartman. (1997). "Exercise training decreases the growth hormone (GH) response to acute constant-load exercise." *Med Sci Sports Exer. May;29(5):660-76.*

Weltman, Pritzlaff, Wideman, Blumer, Abbott, Hartman, Veldhuis. (2000). "Exercise-dependent growth hormone release is linked to markers of heightened central adrenergic outflow." *J Appl Physiol.* Aug;89(2):629-35.

Wideman, Weltman, Patrie. (2000). "Synergy of L-arginine and GHRP-2 stimulation of growth hormone in men and women: modulation by exercise." *Applied Journal of Physiology.* Oct;279(4) R1467-77.

Wideman L, Weltman, Shah, Story, Veldhuis, Weltman A. (1999). "Effects of gender on exercise-induced growth hormone release." *J Appl Physiol.* Sept;87(3):1154-62. PMID: 10484590.

Zhang, Guoyu, Irwin. (2000). "Utilization of preventative medical services in the United States: a comparison between rural and urban populations." *J Rural Health.* Fall;16(4):349-56.

Chapter 2

Booth, Gordon, Carlson, Hamilton. (2000). "Waging war on modern chronic diseases: primary prevention through exercise biology." *J Appl Physiol.* Feb;88(2):774-87. PMID: 10658050.

Calabresi, Ishikawa, Bartolini. (1996). "Somatostatin infusion suppresses GH secretory burst frequency and mass in normal men." *American Journal of Physiology.* Jun;270(6 Pt1):E975-9. PMID: 8764181.

Chein, Vogt, Terry. (1999). "Clinical experiences using a low-dose, high frequency human growth hormone treatment regimen." *Journal of Advancement in Medicine.* 12(3). www.drchein.com.

Colao, Marzullo, Spiezia. (1999). "Effect of growth hormone and insulin like growth factor on prostate diseases: An ultrasonographic and endocrine study in Acromegaly, GH deficiency, and healthy subjects." *J. Clinical Endocrinol Metab.* 84:1986-91.

Corpas, Harman, Blackman. (1993). Human growth hormone and human aging." *Endocrinol Review,* Feb; 14(1):20-39. National Library of Medicine, PubMed: 8491152.

D'Costa, Ingram, Lenham, Sonntag. (1993). "The regulation and mechanism of Action of growth hormone and insulin-like growth factor 1 during normal aging." *Journal of Reproductive Fertil Suppl:*46:87-98. National Library of Science, PubMed abstract: 8636250.

Jenkins. (1999). "Growth hormone and exercise." *Clin Endocrinol (Oxf).* Jun;50(6):683-9. PMID: 10468938.

Kiernan, King, Kraemer, Stefanick, Killen. (2000). "Characteristics of successful dieters: an application of signal detection methodology." *Ann Behav Med.* Winter;20(1):1-6.PMID: 9755345.

Kraemer, Newton. (2000). "Training for muscular power." *Phys Med Rehabil Clin Am.* May11;(2):341-68. PMID: 10810765.

Gibney, Wallace, Spinks. (1999). "The effects of 10 years of recombinant growth hormone (GH) in adult GH-deficient patients." *J Clin Endocrinol Metab.* 84:2596-2602.

Goji, K. (1993). "Pulsatile characteristics of spontaneous growth hormone (GH) concentration profiles in boys evaluated by an ultrasensitive immunoradiometric assay: evidence for ultradian periodicity of GH secretion." *J Clinical Endocrinology Metabolism.* Mar;76(3):667-70.

Jamieson, Dorman, with Valerie Marriott. *(1997). Growth Hormone: Reversing the Aging Process Naturally. The Methuselah Factor.* East Canaan, Connecticut: SAFE GOODS in conjunction with Longevity News Network.

Lieberman, Hoffman. (1997). "The somatopause: should growth hormone deficiency in older people be treated?" *Clinical Geriatric Medicine.* Nov:13(4):671-84. PMID: 9354748.

Nicklas, Ryan, Treuth, Harman, Blackman, Hurley, Rogers. (1995). "Testosterone, growth hormone and IGF-1 responses to Acute and chronic resistive exercise in man aged 55-70 years." *Int Journal Sports Medicine,* Oct;16(7):445-50. National Library of Science, PubMed abstract: 8550252.

Oldenburg, Ann. (2000). "The fountain of youth flows from a needle." *USA Today.* Nov. 14, 2000.

Pfeifer, Verhovec, Zizek. (1999). "Growth hormone treatment reverses early atherosclerotic changes in GH deficient adults." *J Clin Endocrinol Metab.* 84:453-457.

Rudman, Daniel, and colleagues. (1990). "Effects of human growth hormone in men over 60 years old." *New England Journal of Medicine,* Volume, 323, July 5, 1990, Number 1.

Snibson, Bhathal, Adams. (2001). "Overexpressed growth hormone (GH) synergistically promotes carcinogen-initiated liver tumour growth by promoting cellular proliferation in emerging hepatocellular neoplasms in female and male GH-transgenic mice. *Liver.* Apr;21(2):149-58. PMID: 11318985.

Sports Club Association Newsletter, *International Health Racket.* Nov. 2000.

Takala, Ruokonen, Webster. (1999). "Increased mortality associated with growth hormone treatment in critically III adults." *N Eng J Med* 341:785-92.

Toogood, Shalet. (1998). "Aging and growth hormone." *Baillieres Clinical Endocrinology Metabolism,* July: 12 (2):281-96. National Library of Science, PubMed abstract: 10083897.

Toogood, O'Neill, Shalet. (1996). "Beyond the somatopause: growth hormone deficiency in adults over the age of 60 years." *J Clin Endocrinol Metabol.* Feb; 81(2):460-5. National Library of Science, PubMed abstract: 8636250.

Van Buul-Offers, Kooijman. (1998) "The role of growth hormone and insulin-like growth factors in the immune system." *Cell Mol Life Science,* Oct; 54(10): 1083-94. National Library of Science, PubMed abstract: 9817987.

Winer, Shaw, Baumann. (1990). "Basal plasma growth hormone levels in man: new evidence for rhythmicity of growth hormone secretion." *J Clinical Endocrinology Metabolism.* Jun;70(6):1678-86. PMID: 2347901.

Chapter 3

Ames, BN. (2001). "DNA damage from micronutrient deficiencies is likely to be a major cause of cancer." *Mutat Res.* Apr 18;475(1-2):7-20. PMID: 11205149.

Bewaerets, Moorkens, Abs. (1998). "Secretion of growth hormone in patients with chronic fatigue syndrome." *Growth Hormone IGF Res,* April 8, Suppl B: 127-9. Washington, D.C., National Library of Medicine, PMID: 10990147.

Bruls, Crasson, Van Reeth, Legros. (2000). "Melatonin. II. Physiological and therapeutic effects." *Rev Med Liege.* Sept;55(9):862-70. PMID: 11105602.

Carranza-Lira, Garcia. (2000). "Melatonin and climactery." *Med Sci Monit.* Nov-Dec;6(6):1209-12. PMID: 11208481.

Casabiell, Gualillo, Pombo, Dieguez, Casanueva. (1999). "Growth hormone secretagogues: the clinical future." *Horm Res* 1999;51 Suppl 3:29-33. National Library of Science, PubMed abstract: 10592441.

Colgan, Michael. (1993). *Optimum Sports Nutrition, Your Competitive Edge.* New York, NY. Advanced Research Press.

Centers for Disease Control and Prevention. (2000). "Diabetes, A Serious Public Health Problem, AT-A-GLANCE 2000." *Diabetes Public Health Resource.* Atlanta, Georgia. March 9, 2000.

Centers for Disease Control and Prevention. (2000). "CDC: Diabetes, obesity becoming epidemic." *AP News.* January 25,2001. www.Healthcentral.com.

Cox, Cortright, Dohm, Houmard. (1999). "Effect of aging on response to Exercise training in humans: skeletal muscle GLUT-4 and insulin sensitivity." *J Applied Physiology.* June;86(6):2019-25.

El-Khoury, Pereira, Borgonha, Basile-Filho, Beaumier, Wang, Metges, Ajami, Young. (2000). "Twenty-four hour oral tracer studies with L-lysine at a low and intermediate lysine intake in healthy adults." *Am J Clin Nutr.* Jul;72(1):122-30. PMID: 10871570.

Evans, WJ. (2000). "Vitamin E, Vitamin C, and exercise." *Am J Clin Nutr.* Aug;72(2 Suppl):647S-52S. PMID: 10919971.

Field, Coakley, Must, Spadano, Laird, Dietz, Rimm, Colditz. (2001) "Impact of overweight on the risk of developing common chronic diseases during a 10-year period." *Arch Intern Med.* Jul 9;161(13):1581-6. PMID: 11434789.

Holl, Hartman, Veldhuis, Taylor, Thorner. (1991). "Thirty-second sampling of plasma growth hormone in man: correlation with sleep stages." *Journal Clin endocrinol Metab.* Apr;72(4):854-61. PMID: 2005213.

Kami. Hayakawa, Urata, Uchiyama, Shibui, Kim, Kudo, Owawa. (2000). "Melatonin treatment for circadian rhythm sleep disorders." *Psychiatry Clin Neurosci.* Jun;54(3):381-2. PMID: 11186123.

Lanzi, Luzi, Caumo, Andreotti, Manzoni, Malighetti, Sereni, Pontiroli. (1999). "Elevated insulin levels contribute to the reduced growth hormone (GH) response to GH-releasing hormone in obese subjects." *Metabolism,* Sept;48(9):1152-6. PMID: 10484056.

Koo, Huang, Camacho, Trainor, Blake, Sirotina-Meisher, Schleim, Wu, Cheng, Nargund, McKissick. (2001). "Immune enhancing effect of a growth hormone secretagogue." *J Immunol.* Mar 15;166(6):4195-201. PMID: 11238671.

Krzywkowski, Petersen, Ostrowski, Kristensen, Boza, Pedersen. (2001).
    "Effects of glutamine supplementation on exercise-induced changes in
    lymphocyte function." *Am J Physiol Cell Physiol.* Oct;281(4):C1259-65.
    PMID: 11546663.

Marharam, Bauman, Kalman, Skolnik, Perle. (1999). "Masters athletes: factors
    affecting performance." *Sports Med.* Oct;28(4):273-85. PMID: 10565553.

Marcell, Taaffe, Hawkins, Tarpenning, Pyka, Kohlmeier, Wiswell, Marcus. (1999).
    "Oral arginine does not stimulate basal or augment exercise-induced
    GH secretion in either young or old adults." *Journal of Gerontology.*
    A Bio Sci Med Sci. Aug 54(8):M395-9. PMID: 10496544.

Maxwell, Hoai-Ky, Christine, Lin, Bernstein, Cooke. (2001). "L-arginine
    enhances aerobic exercise capacity in association with augmented nitric oxide
    production." *Journal of Applied Physiology; Heart and Circulatory Physiology.*
    March;90(4):933-38.

Momany, Bowers, Reynolds, Chang, Hong, Newlander. (1981). "Design,
    synthesis, and biological activity of peptides which release growth hormone in
    vitro." *Endocrinology.* Jan;108(1):31-9. PMID: 6109621.

Rao, G. (2001). "Insulin resistance syndrome." Am Fam Physician.
    Mar 15;63(6):1159-63, 1165-6. PMID: 11277552.

Reaven, G. (2001). "Syndrome X." *1092-8464* Aug;31(4):323-332. PMID: 11445062.

Robinson, Sloan, Arnold. (2001). "Use of niacin in the prevention and
    management of hyperlipidemia." *Prog Cardiovasc Nurs.* Winter;16(1):14-20.
    PMID: 11252872.

Ryan, Hurlbut, Lott, Ivey, Fleg, Hurley, Goldberg. (2001). "Insulin action after
    resistive training in insulin resistant older men and women."
    J Am Geriatr Soc. Mar;49(3):247-53. PMID: 11300234.

Rubin, Rita. (2001). "More people need cholesterol drugs." *USA Today.* May 16, 2001.

Sanders, Chaturvedi, Hordinski. (1999). "Melatonin: aeromedical,
    toxicopharmacological, and analytical." *J Anal Toxicol.*
    May-Jun;23(3):159-67. PMID: 10369324.

Suminski, Robertson, Goss, Arslamian, Kang, DaSilva, Utter, Metz. (1997)
    "Acute effect of amino acid ingestion and resistance exercise on plasma growth
    hormone concentration in young men." *Int Journal Sports Nutrition,*
    March;7(1):48-60. PMID: 9063764.

Sytze, Smid, Niesink, Bolscher, Waasdorp, Dieguez, Casanueva, Koppeschaar. (2000). "Reduction of free fatty acids by acipimox enhances the growth hormone responses to GH-releasing peptide 2 in elderly men." _J Clin Endocrinol Metab._ Dec;85(12):4706-11. PMID: 11134132.

Tennessee News Service. (2001). "FDA urged to beef up statin warning." _The Tennessean._ Washington / Nation section. August 21, 2001.

Van Cauter, Copinschi. (2000). "Interrelationships between growth hormone and sleep." _Growth Horm IGF Res._ Apr;10 Suppl B:S57-62. PMID: 10984255.

Van Cauter, Leproult, Plat. (2000). "Age-related changes in slow wave and REM sleep and relationship with growth hormone and cortisol levels in healthy men." _JAMA._ Aug 16;284(7):861-8. PMID: 10938176.

Welbourne, TC. (1995). "Increased plasma bicarbonate and growth hormone after an oral glutamine load." _American Journal of Clinical Nutrition,_ Vol.61,1058-1061. National Library of Science, PubMed abstract: 7733028.

Zello, Pencharz, Ball. (1993). "Dietary lysine requirement of young adult males determined by oxidation of L-[1-13C] phenylalanine." _Am J Physiol._ Apr;264(4 Pt1):E677-85. PMID: 8476044.

Chapter 4

Gastin, PB. (2001). "Energy system interaction and relative contribution during maximal exercise." _Sports Med 2001_;31(10):725-41. PMID: 115478894.

Gordon, Kraemer, Vos, Lynch, Knuttgen. (1994). "Effect of acid-base on growth hormone response to acute high-intensity cycle exercise." _J Appl Physiol._ Feb;76(2):821-9. PMID: 8175595.

Hennessey, Chromiak, DellaVentura, Reinert, Puhl, Kiel, Rosen, Vandenburgh, MacLean. (2001). "Growth hormone administration and exercise effects on muscle fiber type and diameter in moderately frail older people." _J AM Geriatr._ Jul:49(7):852-8. PMID: 11527474.

Jesper, Anderson, Schjerling, Saltin. (2000). Muscles, Genes and Athletic Performance." _Scientific American._ Sept(1)48-55.

Kadi, Eriksson, Holmner, Thornell. (1999). "Effects of anabolic steroids on the Muscle cells of strength-trained athletes." _Med Sci Sports Exerc._ Nov;31(11):1528-34. PMID: 10589853.

Lugar, Watschinger, Duester, Svoboda, Clodi. (1992). "Plasma growth hormone and prolactin responses to graded levels of acute exercise and to a lactate infusion. _Neuroendocrinology._ 56;112-117.

Roemmich, Rogol. (1997). "Exercise and growth hormone: does one affect the other?" *J Pediatr.* Jul;131(1 Pt 2):5S75-80. PMID: 9255234.

Vance. (1996.) "Nutrition, body composition, physical activity and growth hormone secretion." *J Pediatr Endocrinol Metab.* Jun;9 Suppl 3:299-301. PMID: 8887174.

VanHelder, Casey, Radomski. (1987). "Regulation of growth hormone during exercise by oxygen demand and availability." *Eur J Appl Physiol Occup Physiol.* 56(6):628-32. PMID: 2678214.

VanHelder, Goode, Radomski. (1984). "Effects of anaerobic and aerobic exercise Of equal duration and work expenditure on plasma growth hormone levels." *Eur J Appl Physiol Occup Physiol.* 52(3):255-7. PMID: 6539675.

Chapter 5

Bell, Syrotuik, Martin, Burnham, Quinney. (2000). "Effect of concurrent strength and endurance training on skeletal muscle properties and hormone concentrations in humans." *Eur J Appl Physiol.* Mar;81(5):418-27. PMID: 10751104.

Evans. (1992). "Exercise, nutrition, and aging." *J Nutr.* Nar;122(3Suppl)796-801. PMID: 1542050.

Hurel, Koppiker, Newkirk, Close, Miller, Mardell, Woos, Kendall-Taylor. (1999). "Relationship pf physical exercise and aging to growth hormone production." *Clin Endocrinol (Oxf).* Dec;51(6):687-91. PMID: 10619972.

Hurrell. (1997). "Factors associated with regular exercise." *Percept Mot Skills.* Jun;84(3Pt 1):871-4. PMID: 9172196.

Jakicic, Winters, Lang, Wing. (1999). "Effects of intermittent exercise and use of home exercise equipment adherence, weight loss, and fitness in overweight women: a random trial." *JAMA.* Oct 27;282(16):1554-60. PMID: 10546695.

Kanaley, Weltman, Pieper, Weltman, Hartman. (2001). "Cortisol and growth Hormone response to exercise at different times of day." *J Clin Endocrinol Metab.* Jun;86(6):2881-9. PMID: 11397904.

Li, Holm, Gulanick, Lanuza, Penckofer. (1999). "The relationship between physical activity and perimenopause." *Health Care Women Int.* Mar-Apr;20(2):163-78. PMID: 10409986.

Rodriguez-Arnao, Jabbar, Fulcher, Besswer, Ross. (1999). "Effects of growth hormone replacement on physical performance and body composition in GH deficient adults." *Clin Endocrinol (Oxf).* Jul;51(1):53-60. PMID: 10468965.

Sesso, Paffenbarger, Lee. (2000). "Physical activity and coronary disease in men: The Harvard Alumni Health Study." _Circulation._ Aug 29;102(9):975-80. PMID: 10961960.

McGuire, Levine, Williamson, Snell, Blomquist, Saltin, Mitchell. (2001). "A 30-year follow-up of the Dallas Bedrest and training Study: II. Effect of age on cardiovascular adaptation to exercise training. _Circulation._ Sept 18;104(12):1358-66. PMID 11560850.

Silverman, Mazzeo. (1996). "Hormonal responses to maximal and submaximal exercise in trained and untrained men of various ages. _J Gerontol A Biol Med Sci._ Jan;51(1):B30-7.

Widrick, Trappe, Costill, Fits. (1996.) "Force-velocity and force- Power properties of single fiber from elite master runners and sedentary med." _Am J Physiol._ Aug;271 (2Pt 1):C676-83.

Chapter 6

Bandy, Irion. (1994). "The effect of time on static stretch on the flexibility of the hamstring muscles." _Phys Ther._ Sept;74(9):845-50. PMID: 8066111.

Dunton, Ross. (2001). _Masters Track and Field News._ Daily email edition, Wednesday, January 17, 2001.

Fowles, Sale, MacDougall. (2000). "Reduced strength after passive stretch of The human plantar flexors." _J Appl Physiol._ Sept;89(3):1179-88.

Hansen, Stevens, Coast. (2001). "Exercise duration and mood state: how much is enough to feel better?" _Health Psychol._ Jul;29(4):267-75. PMID: 11515738

Leach, RE. (2000). "Aging and Physical activity." _Orthopade._ Nov;29(11):936-40. PMID: 11149278.

Magnusson. (1998). "Passive properties of human skeletal muscle during stretch maneuvers." _Scand J Med Sci Sports._ Apr;8(2):65-77. PMID: 9564710.

Manchanda, Narang, Reddy, Sachdeva, Prabhakaran, Dharmanand, Rajani, Bijlani. (2000). _J Assoc Physicians India._ "Retardation of Coronary atherosclerosis with yoga lifestyle intervention." Jul;48:687-94. PMID: 11491594.

Roberts, Wilson. (1999). "Effect of stretching duration on active and passive range of motion in the lower extremity." _Br J Sports Med._ Aug;33(4):259-63. PMID: 10450481.

Tabrizi, McIntryre, Quesnel, Howard. (2000). "Limited dorsiflexion predisposes to injuries of the ankle in children." *J Bone Joint Surg Br.* Nov;82(8):1103-6. PMID: 11132266.

Sothern, Loftin, Udall, Suskind, Ewing, Tang, Blecker. (2000). "Safety, feasibility, and efficacy of a resistance training program in preadolescent obese children." *Am J Med Sci.* Jun;310(6):370-5. PMID: 10875292.

Wang, Whitney, Burdett, Janosky. (1993). "Lower extremity muscular flexibility in long distance runners." *J Orthop Sports Phys Ther.* Feb;17(2):102-7. PMID: 8467336.

Chapter 7

Antonio, Sanders, Ehler, Uelmen, Raether, Stout. (2000). "Effects of exercise training and amino-acid supplementation on body composition and physical performance in untrained women." *Nutrition.* Nov-Dec;16(11-12):1043-6. PMID: 11118822.

Gillespie, Grant. (2000). "Interventions for preventing and treating stress fractures and stress reactions of bone of the lower limbs in young adults." *Cochrane Database Syst Rev 2000.* (2):CD000450. PMID: 10796367.

Kanaley, Weatherup-Dentes, Jaynes, Hartman. (1999). "Obesity attenuates the growth hormone response to exercise." *J Clin Endocrinol Metab.* Sept;84(9):3156-61.

Kraemer, Keuning, Ratamess, Volek. (2001). "Resistance training combined with bench-step aerobics enhances women's health profile." *Med Sci Sports Exerc.* Feb;33(2):259-69. PMID: 11224816.

Marcinik, Potts, Schlabach, Will, Dawson, Hurley. (1991.) "Effects of strength training on lactate thresholds and endurance performance." *Med Sci Sports Exerc.* Jun;23(6):739-43. PMID: 1886483.

Medbo, Tabata. (1989). "Relative importance of aerobic and anaerobic energy Release during short-lasting exhausting bicycle exercise." *J Appl Physiol.* Nov;67(5):1881-6. PMID: 2600022.

Ronsen, Haug, Pedersen, Bahr. (2001). "Increased neuroendocrine response to a repeated bout of endurance exercise." Med Sci Sports Exerc. Apr;33(4):568-75. PMID: 11283432.

Sipila, Elorinne, Alen, Suominen, Kovanen. (1997). "Effects of strength and Endurance training on muscle fiber characteristics in elderly women." *Clin Physiol.* Sept;17(5):459-74. PMID: 9347195.

Sutton, Muir, Mockett, Fentem. (2001). "A case-control study to investigate the relation between low and moderate levels of physical activity and osteoarthritis of the knee using data collected as part of the Allied Dunbar National Fitness Survey." _Ann Rheum Dis._ Aug;60(8):756-64. PMID: 11454639.

Taylor, Bachman. (1999). "The effects of endurance training on muscle fiber types and enzyme activities." _Can J Appl Physiol._ Feb;24(1):41-53. PMID: 9916180.

Chapter 8

Cuneo, Salomon, Wiles, Sonksen. (1990). "Skeletal muscle performance in adults with growth hormone deficiency." _Horm Res._ 33 Suppl 4:66-60. PMID: 2245969.

Dintiman, Ward, Tellez. (1998). _Sports Speed. Second edition._ Champaign, Illinois: Human Kinetics.

Gaskill, Serfass. Bacharach, Kelly. (1999). "Responses to training in cross-country skiers." _Med Sci Sports Exerc._ Aug;31(8):1211-7. PMID: 10449026.

Kindermann, Schnabel, Schmitt, Biro, Cassens, Weber. (1982.) "Catecholamines, growth hormone, cortisol, insulin, and sex hormones in anaerobic and aerobic exercise. _Eur J Appl Occup Physiol._ 49(3):389-99. PMID: 6754371.

Medbo, Burgers. (1990). "Effect of training on the anaerobic capacity." _Med Sci Sports Exerc._ Aug;22(4):501-7. PMID: 2402211.

Mujika, Chatard, Busso, Geyssant, Barale, Lacoste. (1995). "Effects of training on performance in competitive swimming." _Can J Appl Physiol._ Dec;20(4):395-406. PMID: 8563672.

Nevill M, Holmyard, Hall, Allsop, Oosterhout, Burrin, Nevill A. (1996). "Growth hormone responses to treadmill sprinting in sprint- and endurance trained athletes." _Eur J Appl Occup Physiol._ 72(5-6):460-7. PMID: 8925817.

Track & Field News. (2001). Last Lap. "Super Bowl's Track Connection." March p. 49.

Vanhelder, Radomski, Goode, Casey. (1985). "Hormonal and metabolic response to three types of exercise of equal duration and external work output." _Eur J Appl Occup Physiol._ 54(4):337-42. PMID: 3905393.

Chapter 9

Barstow, Jones, Nguyen, Casaburi. (1996). "Influence of muscle fiber and pedal frequency on oxygen uptake and kinetics of Heavy exercise." *J Appl Physiol.* Oct;81(4):1642-50. PMID: 8904581.

Cook, Schultz, Omey, Wolfe, Brunt. (1993). "Development of lower leg strength and flexibility with the strength shoe. *Am J Sports Med.* May-Jun;21(3):445-8. PMID: 8346761.

Fuchs, Bauer, Snow. (2001). "Jumping improves hip and spine and lumbar bone mass in prepubescent children: a randomized controlled trial." *J Bone Miner Res.* Jan ;16(1):148-56. PMID: 11149479.

Kostka, T. (2000). "Physio-pathologic aspects of aging—possible influence of physical training on physical fitness." *Przegl Lek.* 57(9):474-6. PMID: 11199868.

Lemura, Von Duvillard, Mookerjee. (2000). "The effects of physical training on functional capacity in adults. Ages 46 to 90: a meta-analysis." *J Sports Med Phy Fitness.* Mar;40(1):1-10. PMID: 10822903.

Newton, Kraemer, Hakkinen. (1999). "Effects of ballistic training on preseason preparation of elite volleyball players." *Med Sci Sports Exerc.* Feb/31(2):323-30. PMID: 10063823.

Thompson, Glenn. (2001.) "Training Advice." *National Master News.* Feb.270: p.16.

Trappe, Costill, Thomas. (2000). "Effect of swim taper on whole muscle and single muscle fiber contractile properties." *Med Sci Sports Exerc.* Dec;32(12):48-56. PMID: 11224794.

Wheeler, A. (1986). "Isshinryu, one heart - one mind method." *National Paperback Books, Inc.* Knoxville, Tennessee.

Wilson, Murphy, Giorgi. (1996). "Weight and plyometric training; effects on eccentric and concern force production." *Can J Appl Physiol.* Aug;21(4):301-15. PMID: 8853471.

Winters, Snow. (2000). "Detraining reverses positive effects of exercise on the musculoskeletal system in premenopausal women." J Bone Miner Res. Dec;15(12):2495-503. PMID: 11127215.

Witzke, Snow. (2000). "Effects of plyometric jump training on bone mass in adolescent girls." *Med Sci Sports Exerc.* Jun;32(6):1051-7. PMID: 10862529.

Young, Skelton. (1994). "Applied physiology of strength and power in old age." Int J Sports Med. Apr;15(3):149-51. PMID: 8005728.

Chapter 10

American Academy of Pediatrics. (2001). "Strength training by Children and Adolescents (RE0048). 8/29/01. Internet: www.aap.org/policy/re0048.html

Borst, DeHoyos, Garzarella, Vincent, Pollock, Lowenthal. (2001). "Effects of resistance training on insulin-like growth factor-1 and IGF binding proteins." *Med Sci Sports Exerc.* Apr;33(4):648-653. PMID: 11283443.

Bemben DA, Fetters, Bemben MG, Nabavi, Koh. (2000). "Musculoskeletal responses to high- and low–intensity resistance training in early postmenopausal women." *Med Sci Sports Exerc.* Nov;32(11):1949-57. PMID: 11079527

Broeder, Quindry, Brittingham, Panton, Thomson, Appakon, Breuel, Byrd, Douglas, Earnest, Mitchell, Olson, Roy, Yarlaragadda. (2000). "The Andro Project: physiological and hormonal influences of androstenedione supplementation in men 35 to 65 years old participating in a high-intensity resistance training program." *Arch Intern Med.* Nov;13;160(20):3093-104. PMID: 11074738.

Brown, Vukovich, Sharp, Reifenrath, Parson, King. (1999). "Effect of oral DHEA on serum testosterone and adaptations to resistance training in young men." *J Appl Physiol.* Dec;87(6):2274-83. PMID: 10601178.

Cauder, Chilibeck, Webber, Sale. (1994). "Comparison of whole and split weight training routines in young women." *Can J Appli Physiol.* Jun;19(2):185-99. PMID: 8081322.

Escamilla, RF. (2001). "Knee biomechanics of the dynamic squat exercise." *Med Sci Sport Exerc.* Jan;33(1):127-41. PMID: 11194098.

Gibala. (2000). "Nutritional supplementation and resistance exercise: what is the evidence for enhanced skeletal muscle hypertrophy?" *Can J Appl Physiol.* Dec;25(6):524-35. PMID: 11098159.

Hurley, Roth. (2000). "Strength training in elderly: effects on risk factors for age related diseases." *Sports Med.* Oct;30(4):249-268. PMID: 11048773.

Izquierdo, Hakkinen, Ibanez, Anton, Larrion, Gorostiaga. (2001). Effects of strength training on muscle power and serum hormones in middle-aged and older men. *J Appl Physiol.* Abstract-A531-0. Jan. 29,2001.

Joyner. (2000). "Over-the-counter supplements and strength training." *Exerc Sport Sci Rev.* Jan;28(1):2-3. PMID: 11131684.

Kreider. (1999). "Dietary supplements and the promotion of muscle growth with resistance exercise." *Sports Med.* Feb;27(2):97-110. PMID: 10091274.

Jubrias, Esselman, Price, Cress, Conley. (2001). "Large energetic adaptations of elderly muscle to resistance and endurance training. *J Appl Physiol.* Abstract: 8:0057A. Feb. 27, 2001.

Koutedakis, Frischnecht, Murthy. (1997). "Knee flexion to extension peak torque ratios and low-back injuries in highly active individuals." *Int J Sports Med.* May;18(4):290-5. PMID: 9231847.

Mujika, Padilla, Ibanez, Izquierdo, Gorostiaga. (2000). "Creatine supplementation and sprint performance in soccer." *Med Sci Sports Exerc.* Feb;32(2):518-25. PMID: 10694141.

Panton, Rathmacher, Baier, Nissen. (2000). "Nutritional supplementation of the leucine metabolite beta-hydroxy-beta-methylbutyrate (hmb) during resistance training." *Nutrition.* Sep;16(9):734-9. PMID: 10978853.

Pu, Johnson, Forman, Hausdorf, Roubenoff, Foldvari, Feilding, Singh. (2001). "Randomized controlled trial of progressive resistance training to counteract the skeletal muscle myopahthy of chronic heart failure." *J Appl Physiol.* Abstract: 8:0079A. Feb. 27, 2001.

Rennie, MJ. (2001). "Grandad, it ain't what you eat, it depends when you eat it – that's how muscles grow!" *J Physiol.* Aug 15;535(Pt 1):2. PMID: 11507153.

Ross, Dagnone, Jones, Smith, Paddags, Hudson, Janssen, (2000). "Reduction In obesity and related comorbid conditions after diet-induced weight loss or exercise-induced weight loss in Men. A randomized, controlled trial." *Ann Intern Med.* Jul 18;188(2):92-103. PMID: 10896648.

Schilling, Stone, Utter, Kearney, Johnson, Coglianese, Smith, O'Bryant, Fry, Starks, Stone. (2001). "Creatine supplementation and health variables: a retrospective study." *Med Sci Sports Exerc.* Feb;33(2):183-8. PMID: 11224803.

Sothern, Loftin, Udall, Suskind, Ewing, Tang, Blecker. (2000). "Safety, feasibility, and efficacy of a resistance training program in preadolescent obese children." *Am J Med Sci.* Jun;310(6):370-5. PMID: 10875292.

Stone, Sanborn, Smith, O'Bryant, Hoke, Utter, John, Boros, Hruby, Pierce, Stone, Garner. (1999). "Effects of in-season (5-weeks) creatine and pyruvate supplements on anaerobic performance and body composition in American football players." *Int J Sport Nutr.* Jun;9(2):146-65. PMID: 10362452.

Stromme, Hostmark. (2000). "Physical activity, overweight and obesity." *Tidsskr Nor Laegeforen.* Nov 30;120(29):3578-3582. PMID: 11188389.

Wilk, Voight, Keirns, Gambetta, Andrews, Dillman. (1993). "Stretch-shortening drills for the upper extremities: theory and clinical application." *J Orthop Sports Phys Ther.* May;17(5):225-39. PMID: 8343780.

Ahmaidi, Masse-Biron, Adam, Choquet, Freville, Libert. (1998). "Effects of interval training at ventilatory thresholds on clinical and cardiorespiratory responses in elderly humans." *Eur J Appl Physiol Occup Physiol.* Jul;78(2):170-6. PMID: 9694317.

Foster Higgins quote. (1992). "ASO's Feast of Services." *Best's Review,* August 1992. Cited in, "Movement to Self-Insurance Coverage." *Health Care* 1993. *Advisory Board,* August 1997. Washington, D.C.

Mathews, Howard. (1996). "Prescribing Exercise for your patient." *Maryland Medical Journal.* August. #45 (8): 632-7 National Library of Medicine, PMID: 8772277.

McGinnis, Foege. (1993). "Actual Causes of Death in the United States." *JAMA.* 1993. 270:2207-12.

Melillo, Houde, Williamson, Futrell. (2000). "Perceptions of nurse practioners regarding their role in physical activity and exercise prescription for older adults." *Clinical Excellence for Nurse Practitioners.* March 4, (2): 108-16. National Library of Medicine, PMID: 11075052.

O'Brien, S. (2000). "My heart couldn't take it": older women's beliefs about Exercise benefits and risks." *J Gerontol B Psychol Sci Soc Sci.* Sep;55(5):P283-94. PMID: 10985293.

O'Grady, Fletcher, Ortiz. (2000). Therapeutic and physical fitness exercise Prescription for older adults with joint disease: an evidence-based approach." *Rheumatoid Disease North American.* August: 26(3): 617-46. National Library of Medicine. PMID: 10989515.

Conclusion

Desaphy, De Luca, Pierno, Imbrici, Camerino. (1998). "Partial recovery of skeletal muscle sodium channel properties in aged rats chronically treated with growth hormone or the GH secretagogue hexarelin." *J Pharmacol Exp Ther.* Aug;286(2):903-12. PMID: 9694949.

Godin, Shephard. (1990). "Use of attitude-behavior models in exercise promotion." *Sports Med.* Aug;10(2):103-21. PMID: 2204097.

Huddy, Herbert, Hymer, Johnson. (1995). "Facilitating changes in exercise behavior: effect of structured statements of intention on perceived barriers to action." *Psychol Rep.* Jun;73(3 Pt 1):867-76. PMID: 756803.

Lexell, J. (1999). "Effects of strength and endurance training on skeletal muscles in the elderly. New muscles for old!" *Lakartidningen.* Jan 20;96(3):207-9. PMID: 10068322.

Morley, Baumgarter, Roubenoff, Mayer, Nair. (2001). "Sarcopenia."
J Lab Clin Med. Apr;137(4):231-43. PMID: 11283518.

Proctor, Sunning, Walro, Sieck, Lemon. (1995). " Oxidative capacity of human
muscle fiber types: effects of age and training status." *J Appl Physiol.*
Jun;78(6):2033-8. PMID: 7665396.

Trappe, Williamson, Godard, Porter, Rowden, Costill. (2000). "Effect of
resistance training on single muscle fiber contractile function in older men."
J Appl Physiol. Jul;89(1):143-52. PMID: 10904046.

Turner, Wang, Westerfield. (1995). "Preventing release in weight control: a
discussion of cognitive and behavioral strategies." Psychol Rep.
Oct;77(2):651-66. PMID: 8559896.

Glossary

Aerobic Exercise - Exercise that allows your body to consistently replenish its need for oxygen during fitness training. It is performed at a low to moderate intensity for 20 to 30 minutes. Aerobic exercise is frequently called "cardio" and is used to build endurance and cardiovascular conditioning.

Amino Acids - The building blocks of proteins, which build and repair the body.

Anabolic - Growth oriented. The building-up cycle of the human body. Opposed to catabolic, the breaking-down of body tissue.

Anaerobic Exercise - The short, fast high-intensity type of exercise that uses oxygen faster than the body can replenish it.

Antioxidants - Compounds that lessen tissue oxidation and damage to the body. These small compounds assist in controlling potentially damaging free radical cells.

ATP - A high-energy molecule that provides energy to the body at the cellular level.

Atrophy - The loss and wasting of muscle due to inactivity.

Barbell - A long bar, approximately six feet in length that can accommodate weighted plates on each end. The Olympic barbell is the industry standard for heavy lifting.

Carbs / Carbohydrates – Nutrients supplying energy to the body expressed as "simple" (sugar), and "complex" (grains).

Catecholamines – Natural hormones produced by the body (adrenaline and norepinephrine). The body's release of "Catecholamines" during exercise is a growth hormone release benchmark.

Circuit Training - A series of exercises set in sequence. The exercises are performed one after the other, and typically target different muscle groups.

Concentric - The lifting phase when the muscle shortens or contracts. The "positive" movement of an exercise opposed to the "negative" eccentric lengthening phase.

Contraction – Movement of a muscle that results in shortening a muscle to push or pull resistance.

Cool down – The gradual slowing down of heart rate and body temperature that occurs between exercise and normal functioning of the body.

Cross training – The process of using several types of exercise in fitness training.

Dehydration – Losing too much body fluid during training. This can become dangerous if the body does not get replenished with adequate fluid during training. Dehydration will interfere with the release of growth hormone during exercise.

Dorsiflexion - Bending the foot backward (up) during running to gain power from increased ankle action. Opposite of plantarflexion (foot down).

Drop Set – Sometimes called "Giant Set" is a series of three or more exercises performed in succession without rest between sets.

Dumbbell - A shortened version of a barbell, usually measuring about 12 inches in length, that allows an exercise to be performed one arm at a time.

Eccentric - The lowering phase when the muscle lengthens. The "negative" movement of an exercise.

Endorphins – A natural chemical released by the body during training. Endorphins are released by the pituitary gland and act on the nervous system to reduce sensitivity to pain.

Endurance – The ability to perform exercise for an extended period.

Exercise – Prescribed body movements intended to develop the body by working muscle groups.

Exhaustion Principle – A fundamental principle of Synergy Fitness, this is the point in exercise where you cannot physically perform another repetition.

EZ-curl bar - A specially configured barbell that has two sets of curves in the middle in order to reduce strain on the wrist joints.

Fat – An essential nutrient that is a source of energy for the body.

Fatigue - The point in exercise where the muscle begins to weaken.

Flexibility – The degree of muscle and connective tissue attached to joints to move in a full range of motion. Flexibility is increased through stretching.

Free Weights - Barbells and dumbbells.

Glucose – A "simple" sugar used by the body for energy.

Glutamine - An amino acid proven to be effective in increasing growth hormone naturally.

Glycogen – Substance formed by carbohydrates and stored in the body as an energy source.

Growth Hormone (GH) – A hormone produced by the pituitary gland responsible for promoting and regulating muscle and tissue growth, regulating carbohydrates and fat metabolism, and controlling other vital glands.

HDL Cholesterol - High-density lipoprotein. Also known as "good" cholesterol because it has scavenger abilities to remove fats in the blood. Exercise can increase HDL.

Hydration – Drinking fluids.

Hypertrophy - An increase in muscle size.

Hypoglycemia – low blood sugar.

Intensity - The amount of stress on the body while performing an exercise.

Isolation Principle - A fundamental principle of Synergy Fitness. This is the correct positioning of your body that allows one muscle group to be the primary target of an exercise.

Lactic Acid – The natural by-product produced by the body during anaerobic exercise. Lactic acid production in the muscles during exercise is the body's way of telling the muscles that there is not enough oxygen in the blood. The muscles begin producing pain sensations in a direct relationship to the amount of lactic acid produced. This is a GH-release benchmark.

Lateral - To the side.

LDL Cholesterol - Low-density lipoprotein. Considered "bad" cholesterol due to its negative impact on the cardiovascular system.

Metabolism - The chemical reactions that occur in the body. "Metabolic rate" is the rate at which the body utilizes energy. Exercise increases metabolic rate.

Muscle Pump - The pooling of blood in a muscle during exercise.

Muscle Tone - The condition of muscle that appears healthy and firm.

Nutrients - Nourishment for the body. Macronutrients are carbohydrates, protein, fat and water. Micronutrients are vitamins and minerals. "Essential nutrients" must be obtained from the diet.

Obesity - Over 30 percent body fat.

Peptides - Two or more amino acids linked together.

Periodization – A training method that varies training to prepare an athlete to achieve "peak" performance at the prescribed time.

Placebo - A fake treatment used to test research experiments.

Plateau – The halting or leveling off of gains in fitness and training.

Protein – The building block nutrients promoting positive growth and repair of body tissue. Proteins are composed of amino acids.

Recovery – Recovery has two meanings in fitness. (1) During training, "recovery" is the brief period between sets generally lasing one to two minutes. (2) Recovery is the period immediately following training typically lasting 30 minutes.

Repetition (Rep) - One complete movement of an exercise.

Resistance - The amount of weight or force used in an exercise.

Routine - The configuration of exercises - sets and reps - utilized in fitness training.

Set - A series of repetitions. Example: "2 sets of 10 repetitions."

Somatostatin – A hormone that inhibits the release of growth hormone.

Static Stretching - Holding a stretching position without movement.

Strength training – Exercise to increase strength; weightlifting, resistance training.

Superset - Two exercises performed in succession with little or no rest between sets.

Symmetry - The way muscle groups appear to compliment one another, creating a proportional physique.

Synergistic - Parts working together and producing more together than individual parts would produce alone.

Technique – The form utilized in performing the biomechanics of an exercise.

Warm-up – slow and mild exercise that seeks to raise body temperature by one degree prior to fitness training.

Whey Protein - Protein and protein supplements that are made from milk.

Index

L

Lysine 62

M

Masters Track and Field 164
Melatonin Supplements 56
Moving Plyometrics 175
Muscle Burn 31
Muscle Fiber Activation 93
Muscle Fiber Composition 92
Muscle Fiber Types 88
Muscle Memory 105

N

Negative Foot Speed 163
New Fitness Paradigm 338
Niacin 63

O

Over-Speed Training 158
Oxygen Deficit 30

P

Personal Trainer Resources 209
Plyo-Lifts 185
Plyo-Power 167
Plyo-Weight Training 181
Plyometric Drills 169-175
Plyometrics 168
Protein Supplements 210

R

Repetition Tempo 202
Reps 198
Resistance Routines 203
Resistance Training Supplements 210
Resistance Training Principles 195
Road Running 141

S

T

U

QUICK ORDER FORM

Ready, Set, GO! Synergy Fitness for Time-Crunched Adults

FREE SHIPPING on 2 or More Books!

Name _____

Address _____

City _____

State_____ Zip _____Country_____

___YES! Please rush Ready, Set, GO! in the following quantities:

_____Copies x $19.95   = $ _____

SHIPPING: 1 book shipping @ $3.00   = $ _____

2 or more books in the U.S.   = $ __FREE__

TN residents add 8.75% sales   = $ _____

tax   = $ _____

ORDER TOTAL:

(Please pay in U.S. funds)

Check Enclosed ____   MasterCard____   Visa____   Discover____

Card # _____

Exp. Date _____

Signature _____

Mail to: Pristine Publishers Inc. USA
833 Grayson Lane
Jackson, TN 38305

Orders: www.readysetgofitness.com   *Email:* pristine@charter.net
Toll Free: 1 (866) 565-3311   *Fax orders:* 1 (954) 212-0512

QUICK ORDER FORM

Ready, Set, GO! Synergy Fitness for Time-Crunched Adults

FREE SHIPPING on 2 or More Books!

Name _____

Address _____

City _____

State_____ Zip _____Country_____

____**YES! Please rush Ready, Set, GO! in the following quantities:**

_____Copies x $19.95   = $ _____

SHIPPING: 1 book shipping @ $3.00   = $ _____
                        2 or more books in the U.S.   = $ **FREE**
                        TN residents add 8.75% sales = $ _____
tax   = $ _____
                              ORDER TOTAL:
                       (Please pay in U.S. funds)

Check Enclosed ____   MasterCard____   Visa____   Discover____
Card # _____
Exp. Date _____
Signature _____

Mail to: Pristine Publishers Inc. USA
            833 Grayson Lane
            Jackson, TN 38305

Orders: www.readysetgofitness.com   *Email:* pristine@charter.net
Toll Free: 1 (866) 565-3311   *Fax orders:* 1 (954) 212-0512